Public Health and Epidemiology at a Glance

Margaret Somerville

MD, MRCP, FFPH
Director of Public Health and Health Policy
NHS Highland
Inverness, UK

K. Kumaran

DM, FFPH
Consultant in Public Health Medicine
NHS Somerset
Somerset, UK

Rob Anderson

PhD, MSc, MA(Econ.)
Peninsula Technology Assessment Group (PenTAG)
Institute of Health Service Research
Peninsula Medical School
Exeter, UK

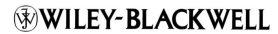
WILEY-BLACKWELL

A John Wiley & Sons, Ltd., Publication

This edition first published 2012 © 2012 by John Wiley & Sons, Ltd.

Wiley-Blackwell is an imprint of John Wiley & Sons, formed by the merger of Wiley's global Scientific, Technical and Medical business with Blackwell Publishing.

Registered office: John Wiley & Sons, Ltd, The Atrium, Southern Gate, Chichester, West Sussex, PO19 8SQ, UK

Editorial offices: 9600 Garsington Road, Oxford, OX4 2DQ, UK
The Atrium, Southern Gate, Chichester, West Sussex, PO19 8SQ, UK
111 River Street, Hoboken, NJ 07030-5774, USA

For details of our global editorial offices, for customer services and for information about how to apply for permission to reuse the copyright material in this book please see our website at www. wiley.com/wiley-blackwell.

Library of Congress Cataloging-in-Publication Data

Somerville, Margaret, Dr.
  Public health and epidemiology at a glance / Margaret Somerville, Kalyanaraman Kumaran, Robert Anderson.
      p. ; cm. – (At a glance)
  Includes bibliographical references and index.
  ISBN-13: 978-0-470-65445-3 (pbk. : alk. paper)
  ISBN-10: 0-470-65445-7 (pbk. : alk. paper)
  I. Kumaran, Kalyanaraman. II. Anderson, Robert, 1967- III. Title. IV. Series: At a glance series (Oxford, England).
  [DNLM: 1. Epidemiologic Methods. 2. Public Health. 3. Needs Assessment. WA 105]
  LC classification not assigned
  614.4–dc23
                                    2011028910

A catalogue record for this book is available from the British Library.

Wiley also publishes its books in a variety of electronic formats. Some content that appears in print may not be available in electronic books.

Set in 9 on 11.5 pt Times by Toppan Best-set Premedia Limited
Printed and bound in Malaysia by Vivar Printing Sdn Bhd

1   2012

Public Health and Epidemiology
at a Glance

Contents

Preface

This book has arisen from our experience of developing a new undergraduate medical course for the Peninsula Medical School. In the early days, we were conscious of staying just one step ahead of the students in terms of planning the next stage of the curriculum. Now that the course is well-established, we are inevitably reflecting on where and how in the curriculum public health and epidemiology are best delivered. The GMC guidance in *Tomorrow's Doctors* stresses the fundamental importance of public health as a core element of medical training; consequently our considered view is that learning about public health principles and practice should be fully integrated into all aspects of clinical learning.

Another important principle is that students should learn from people working in service public health, just as they learn from active clinicians in other fields. We have tried to ensure that this book covers public health topics, and particularly epidemiology, in such a way that the practical applications of theory and principles to public health service work can be seen. We would recommend that students whose interest is sparked by this book should actively seek out public health professionals (who can be found in many different places, not just the health service) to find out about their everyday work.

Margaret Somerville MD, MRCP, FFPH
K. Kumaran DM, FFPH
Rob Anderson PhD, MSc, MA(Econ.)

Acknowledgements

We had the support and guidance of many people in developing the Peninsula Medical School course and we have used much of the material as the basis for the chapters in this book, but we would particularly like to thank Stuart Paynter, Graham Taylor, Stuart Logan and Ken Stein for their help with parts of the curriculum relating to epidemiology, evidence-based practice and statistics. Any misrepresentation of their original contributions to the teaching material is entirely our responsibility.

We are also very grateful for the help and guidance from Wiley-Blackwell, particularly Laura Murphy and Elizabeth Johnston, in getting this book from ideas to finished product.

About the authors

Margaret Somerville

Margaret Somerville is Director of Public Health and Health Policy for NHS Highland, a post she took up in 2010. Previously, she was Director of Public Health Learning at the Peninsula Medical School, where she developed the public health aspects of the integrated undergraduate medical curriculum from the outset of the course in 2002.

K. Kumaran

Kumaran is a Consultant in Communicable Disease Control at the South West (South) Health Protection Unit and a Consultant in Public Health at NHS Somerset. He also holds an honorary academic post as Clinical Lecturer at the Peninsula Medical School. Previously, in his substantive part-time role at the medical school, he was involved in the development and delivery of the undergraduate public health curriculum between 2004 and 2010 working with other colleagues.

Rob Anderson

Rob Anderson is Associate Professor of Health Economics and Evaluation within the Peninsula Medical School, at the University of Exeter. With others, he has developed and taught the health economics and related components of the undergraduate medical curriculum at the medical school since 2005. His research involves the evaluation and economic evaluation of health technologies and public health policies and programmes to inform national policy.

1 Introduction to public health

(a) An illustration of the 'downstream' approach of health care services in rescuing people who have fallen into the river, instead of moving 'upstream' to find out why people have fallen in

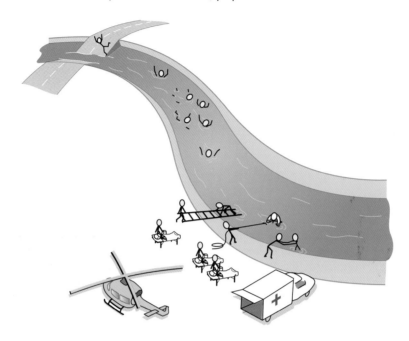

(b) The UK Faculty of Public Health's domains of public health

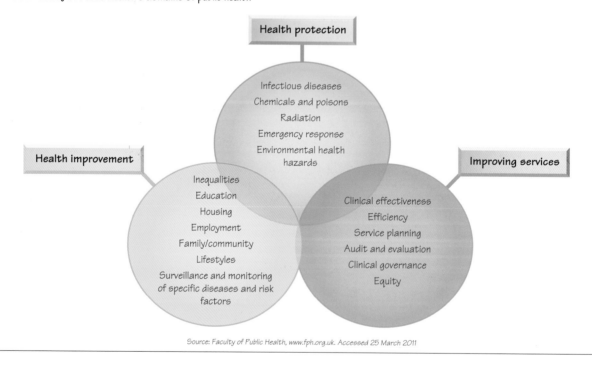

Health protection
- Infectious diseases
- Chemicals and poisons
- Radiation
- Emergency response
- Environmental health hazards

Health improvement
- Inequalities
- Education
- Housing
- Employment
- Family/community
- Lifestyles
- Surveillance and monitoring of specific diseases and risk factors

Improving services
- Clinical effectiveness
- Efficiency
- Service planning
- Audit and evaluation
- Clinical governance
- Equity

Source: Faculty of Public Health, www.fph.org.uk. Accessed 25 March 2011

Public Health and Epidemiology at a Glance, First Edition. Margaret Somerville, K. Kumaran, Rob Anderson.

What is public health? Why do I need to study it? We hear this question a lot from medical students just starting out on their medical careers. There is, of course, the standard definition:

Public health is the science and art of preventing disease, promoting health and well-being and prolonging life through the organised efforts of society (Faculty of Public Health)

. . . but what does this really mean?

The difference between the clinical and public health roles of doctors (and health services) is often illustrated by the image of people pulling others out of a river (Figure 1a). So busy are these people with saving those who are drowning that nobody has thought to go back upstream to find out why people are falling in to begin with. Public health aims to go upstream to find out why people are drowning. As well as understanding the problem, public health also tries to prevent it or reduce the harm resulting from it. Such action may involve persuading decision-makers to put up effective barriers to stop people falling into the river, repairing damaged river banks or controlling flooding, as well as providing information in the right way to prevent risky behaviour near the river. It may also be appropriate to make sure that the people saving those who are drowning are well trained and at the right place on the river bank to save as many lives as possible effectively and efficiently.

Doctors and other health care professionals spend their time dealing with people with health problems – those drowning people – and in treating individuals as effectively as possible. But many individuals' ability to obtain and follow medical advice is limited by circumstances outside their control. They may not be able to get to a clinic or hospital or afford the tests, drugs or other treatment once there; they may not understand the advice or treatment because of educational, language or cultural barriers, or may find it impossible to follow because of their domestic or social circumstances. Understanding these 'upstream' determinants of health is vital to providing health services that are sensitive to people's needs and effective in improving health. Methods of addressing them include legislation (e.g. wearing seat belts or motorcycle helmets), fiscal policy (e.g. taxing alcohol and tobacco), local and national social initiatives (e.g. literacy programmes, housing improvements and cycle paths) as well as more specific disease prevention programmes (e.g. immunisation). Taking such action requires a very different approach to that of the traditional healer, one that recognises that doctors and health care professionals may not be able to act directly themselves, but can work with and influence others to take action to improve health. It involves working with many different people, professionals, organisations and communities both within and outside the health sector.

There can be tensions between the traditional clinical approach to individuals' health problems and this population approach: what leads to improvement in the health of a population as a whole may not mean health improvement for every individual within it.

Conversely, doing what is clinically best for the individual patient may mean others are excluded from getting appropriate, or even any, health care. Getting this balance as right as possible is a public health concern.

So public health is not just about acquiring a detailed knowledge base or a specific set of skills; it is also about an approach to health and health problems that is population-based, rational, transparent and fair. The public health approach seeks to identify and quantify health problems at a population or community level and then develop, introduce and evaluate interventions to improve health, monitoring progress to see whether the actions have made a difference. Epidemiology, the study of disease patterns, is the key discipline that helps us to understand population health, but in order to fulfil the role set out in the previous sentence, public health needs to draw on a wide range of other disciplines and knowledge. Statistics, sociology, psychology, health economics, health promotion, management and leadership, health systems and policy all contribute to the public health approach. This book attempts to give you an introduction to this complex and fascinating subject, which is fundamental to the good practice of medicine.

Domains of public health

The scope of public health, as described above, is very wide-ranging, but is generally recognised as falling into three domains (Figure 1b). All three domains draw on the academic disciplines listed above and all collect or make use of information relevant to health, such as population data from the census, data on health service use (e.g. prescribed drugs, hospital admissions or consultations with health professionals), registrations of births and deaths and disease and risk factor prevalence levels (e.g. alcohol consumption or diabetes).

• **Health protection** covers communicable diseases and environmental hazards, such as exposure to toxic chemicals and poisons. Exposure to hazardous substances at work is covered by the separate discipline of occupational medicine.

• **Health improvement** includes understanding the wider determinants of health, such as housing, education, poverty and lifestyle risk factors and seeks to improve health through health promotion and disease prevention.

• **Improving services** is concerned with how the quality of health services can be improved through evidence-based planning, the provision of effective and cost-effective treatment and ensuring that services are available to everyone who can benefit from them.

In the first section of this book (Chapters 2–11), we cover the main epidemiological concepts and methods that underpin evidence-based practice, whether public health or clinically focussed. The second section (Chapters 12–21) covers the types and sources of information used to assess population health status and need for healthcare. The third section (Chapters 22–30) covers health improvement and the final two sections health economics (Chapters 31–34) and health services (Chapters 35–37).

2 **Incidence and prevalence**

(a) Incidence is represented by new cases of disease (blue) being added to the population. Prevalence is represented by cases of disease (purple) already existing in the population (red)

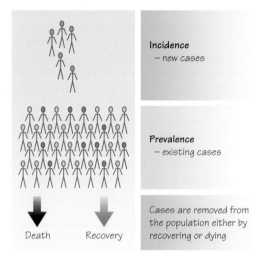

Incidence
– new cases

Prevalence
– existing cases

Death   Recovery

Cases are removed from the population either by recovering or dying

(b) Each horizontal bar represents an individual. The blue section indicates the time spent in good health and the green section time spent with disease. Note that the total time that the individuals have been under observation is 46 years, made up of 8 individuals under observation for 5 years, one under observation for 3.5 years and one under observation for 2.5 years, a total of 46 person-years of observation

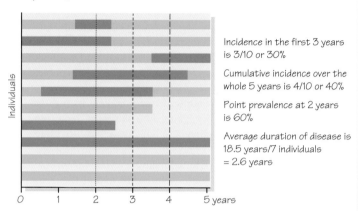

Incidence in the first 3 years is 3/10 or 30%

Cumulative incidence over the whole 5 years is 4/10 or 40%

Point prevalence at 2 years is 60%

Average duration of disease is 18.5 years/7 individuals = 2.6 years

(c) Average annual male mesothelioma death rates per million by age and time period 1970–2005

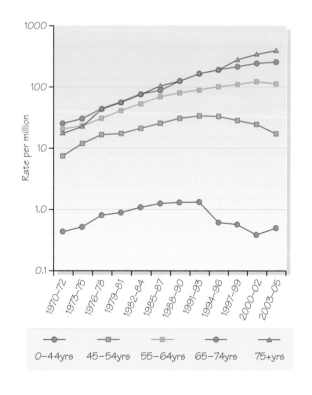

Legend: 0–44yrs   45–54yrs   55–64yrs   65–74yrs   75+yrs

Source: Mesothelioma Mortality in Great Britain: Analyses by Geographical Area and Occupation 2005 (Health and Safety Executive, www.hse.gov.uk)

(d) Mesothelioma mortality by geographical area (2005)

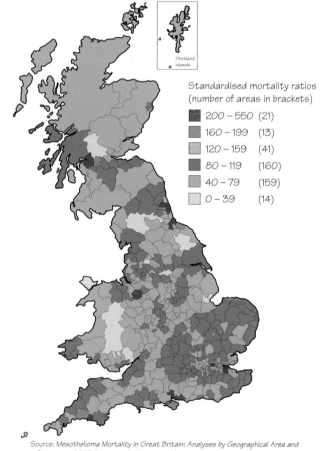

Standardised mortality ratios (number of areas in brackets)

- 200 – 550   (21)
- 160 – 199   (13)
- 120 – 159   (41)
- 80 – 119   (160)
- 40 – 79   (159)
- 0 – 39   (14)

Source: Mesothelioma Mortality in Great Britain: Analyses by Geographical Area and Occupation 2005 (contains public sector information published by the Health and Safety Executive and licensed under the Open Government Licence v1.0')

Public Health and Epidemiology at a Glance, First Edition. Margaret Somerville, K. Kumaran, Rob Anderson.

Definitions

Epidemiology: the study of the occurrence and distribution of health-related states or events in specified populations, including the study of the determinants influencing such states, and the application of this knowledge to control the health problems

Incidence (I): the number of instances of illness commencing, or of persons falling ill, during a given period in a specified population; more generally, the number of new health-related events in a defined population within a specified period of time. It may be measured as a frequency count, a rate or a proportion.

Prevalence (P): the total number of individuals who have an attribute or disease divided by the population at risk of having that attribute or disease either (a) at a specified time (point prevalence), or (b) over a specified period (annual, lifetime, one year) (period prevalence).

(All the above definitions come from M. Porta and J.M. Last, *Dictionary of Epidemiology*, 5th edition, OUP, 2008).

The relationship between incidence and prevalence is modified by the duration of the disease:

$$\text{Prevalence} = \text{incidence} \times \text{duration}$$

High prevalence may result from a high incidence or a long disease duration or both. For example, suppose that in a population of 100 people, 5 new cases of disease occur during the first year of observation (Figure 2a). Assuming that no one in the population had the disease at the start of our observation period, both the prevalence of the disease in the first year and the annual incidence is 5 per 100 people or 5%. If the disease lasts 10 years or more, but no more new cases arise during our second year of observation, then the incidence in the second year is zero, but the prevalence at the end of that time is still 5%.

In Figure 2b, each horizontal bar represents one individual followed over time. The blue section indicates when they have had a particular illness; the green section indicates when they have been well. We can see that two individuals have been well throughout the whole 5-year period that this group has been under observation, while another has also been well for the 3.5 years that he/she has been under observation. One person has been ill for the whole period and another has been ill and then lost to follow-up, or has died, at 2.5 years. Four people developed the illness over the 5-year period, giving us a cumulative incidence over the 5 years of 40%. The seven individuals who were ill during the whole 5-year observation period had a total of 18.5 years of illness, giving us an average duration of disease of 2.6 years.

Rates

Incidence and point prevalence, as used in Figure 2b, are expressed as proportions (percentages), although they were originally expressed as numbers of new and existing cases. In order to express incidence and prevalence as rates, however, the denominator needs to take into account both the number of individuals and the length of time each has been under observation. In Figure 2b, incidence at 3 years is given by the number of new cases arising in the 3-year period (3) divided by the time the individuals have been under observation (29.5 years), giving us an incidence of 10.2 cases per 100 person-years of observation. The period prevalence for years 2–4 is given by the number of prevalent cases (7) divided by the length of time that all individuals were under observation during that time (18 years) giving us a period prevalence of 38.9 cases per 100 person-years of observation. Point prevalence is always expressed as a proportion, as there is no duration of observation to take into account.

The terms incidence and prevalence are frequently used loosely to refer to proportions, rates or numbers, as indicated in the definitions above.

Descriptive epidemiology

Conventionally, incidence and prevalence are described by time, place and person. Figure 2c shows that mesothelioma death rates in men are much higher and increasing in older age groups (men aged 65–74 years and over 75 years), but have been declining at younger ages since around 1990. The map in Figure 2d shows the geographical distribution of mesothelioma deaths in men from 1981–2005 as the standardised mortality ratios (SMRs, see Chapter 6) for men by local and unitary authorities in Great Britain. The areas with the highest SMRs are shown in shades of pink to red.

Describing prevalence and mortality in this way can suggest possible explanations for the observed disease patterns in time, place and person. Hypotheses generated in this way can then be investigated further with specific studies.

3 Risks and odds

Box 3.1 Risk, relative risk and risk difference

- Risk = Number of events ÷ Total population at risk
- Relative risk = Risk in group 1 ÷ Risk in group 2
- Risk difference = Risk in group 1 - Risk in group 2

Note: Risk and risk difference are also referred to as absolute risk and absolute risk difference.

Box 3.2 Risk of seasonal flu in staff and students at a medical school

Risk in staff and students = 150 ÷ 1500 = 10%
Risk in students = 50 ÷ 1000 = 5%
Risk in staff = 100 ÷ 500 = 20%
The risks in the two groups can be compared by two methods:

- Divide the risk in one group by the other, i.e. relative risk:

Relative risk = Risk in staff ÷ Risk in students = 20% ÷ 5% = 4
This implies staff are four times more likely to develop seasonal flu compared with students.

- Subtract the risk in one group from the other, i.e. absolute risk difference:

Absolute risk difference = 20% - 5% = 15%
This implies that for every 100 staff members, there will be 15 extra cases of seasonal flu compared with students.

Box 3.3 Differences between relative risk and absolute risk difference

Hypothetical study examining risk of leukaemia and exposure to benzene	Hypothetical study examining risk of lung cancer and exposure to smoking
Relative risk = 40/1000 ÷ 10/1000 = 4 i.e. those exposed to benzene have 4 times the risk of developing leukaemia as those not exposed to benzene Absolute risk difference = 4% - 1% = 3% i.e. for every 100 people exposed to benzene, there will be 3 extra cases of leukaemia	Relative risk = 80/100 ÷ 20/100 = 4 i.e. those exposed to smoking have 4 times the risk of developing lung cancer as those not exposed to smoking Absolute risk difference = 80% - 20% = 60% i.e. for every 100 people exposed to smoking there will be 60 extra cases of lung cancer.

Box 3.4 Concept of odds

The concept of odds is commonly used by bookmakers in gambling. For example, assume that 20 horses are running in this year's Grand National. If you back a particular horse to win, your horse can only win it if the other 19 horses lose (we exclude the probability of joint winners for this example). Therefore the odds of your horse winning is: the likelihood of your horse winning divided by the likelihood of the other horses winning, i.e. 1/19. The odds against your horse winning is the reverse, i.e. 19/1.
In theory, the bookmakers should therefore offer odds of 19/1 against any horse winning; however, in practice the odds vary because of practical issues such as previous performance, the weight the horse is carrying, and the quality of the trainer and the jockey.

Box 3.5 Calculation of odds and odds ratio

The results of a hypothetical case-control study performed on 100 cases of lung cancer and 100 controls show that 90 of the cases and 30 of the controls have a history of smoking.

	Lung cancer	No lung cancer	Total
Smokers	90	30	100
Non-smokers	10	70	100
Total	100	100	

Odds of smoking in those with lung cancer = 90/10
Odds of smoking in those without lung cancer = 30/70
Odds ratio = 90/10 ÷ 30/70 = 21
i.e. those with lung cancer are more likely to smoke than those without lung cancer.

(Note that the odds ratio has no real numerical significance, i.e. an odds ratio of 21 does not imply those with lung cancer are 21 times more likely to be smokers than those without lung cancer. The further the odds ratio is from 1, the more likely it is that those with the disease have the exposure compared to those without the disease.)

Public Health and Epidemiology at a Glance, First Edition. Margaret Somerville, K. Kumaran, Rob Anderson.

In this chapter, we will look at the main statistical measures used to quantify risk in epidemiological studies.

Risk, relative risk and absolute risk difference

A risk is defined as the number of events divided by the total population at risk over a given time period (Box 3.1).

For example, if there are 150 cases of seasonal flu occurring in 1500 staff and students at the medical school in a year, the risk of a staff or student developing seasonal flu during the academic year 2009–10 is:

Number of cases of flu ÷ Total number of staff and students
= 150 ÷ 1500 = 10%

In epidemiology, useful information is obtained by comparing two groups. Extending the above example, let us assume that there are 1000 students in the school of whom 50 develop seasonal flu. Therefore the risk of students developing flu during the year is 50 ÷ 1000, i.e. 5% (or 0.05 as a proportion). If 100 of 500 staff develop flu, the risk of staff developing flu is 100 ÷ 500, i.e. 20% or 0.2. How can we compare the risks in these two groups? Box 3.2 illustrates two methods of comparing risks in these two groups.

Although there are technical differences, and purists may not agree, in practice relative risk is commonly used as an umbrella term to describe risk ratio and rate ratio. While both relative risk and absolute risk difference are useful to compare two groups, the absolute difference takes into account how common the underlying condition is (i.e. its prevalence) in the population. It has important implications for practice as illustrated by the following hypothetical example.

Example

In a hypothetical study examining the risk of developing leukaemia among those exposed and unexposed to benzene, assume that there were 40 cases of leukaemia in 1000 people exposed to benzene and 10 cases in 1000 people who were unexposed to benzene.

In another scenario examining the risk of developing lung cancer in smokers and non-smokers, there were 80 cases of lung cancer in 100 smokers who were followed up and 20 cases in 100 non-smokers.

Box 3.3 compares the relative and absolute risks in these two scenarios. Here we have two scenarios with identical relative risks – the risk of disease in the group exposed to a risk factor under investigation is four times that of the unexposed group. However, the absolute risk differences are very different – only 3% for benzene and leukaemia and 60% for smoking and lung cancer. This is because lung cancer is more prevalent in the underlying population than is leukaemia, and the absolute risk difference takes that into account. If we therefore had to choose one of these diseases to tackle, we would gain more benefit in public health terms by focusing on stopping people smoking than on preventing exposure to benzene.

Rates are similar to risks, except that the rate takes into account the amount of time each person in the study was at risk for (see Chapter 2).

Odds and odds ratio

Odds is the number of events divided by the number of non-events. Box 3.4 illustrates the concept and its calculation. Mathematically, the difference between odds and risk is illustrated by defining odds as

probability of event ÷ (1 − probability of event)

while risk is just the probability of the event.

Note that if the odds of any event occurring is greater than 1, it implies that the event is more likely to happen than not happen.

In epidemiology, the **odds ratio** is another measure of effect that allows us to compare risk between two groups. It refers to the odds of exposure in one group divided by the odds of exposure in the other group. Relative risks (rate ratios or risk ratios) are preferable to odds ratios as they allow the calculation of the risk of developing the condition unlike odds ratios.

Consider an example looking at smoking as a risk factor for lung cancer (Box 3.5). Odds ratios are most useful in case-control studies in which absolute risks cannot be calculated (except in very rare circumstances, the discussion of which is beyond the scope of this book). Odds ratios approximate to risk ratios when a disease is rare and hence are useful in case-control studies. Although odds ratios can also be used in cohort studies or randomised controlled trials, measures of relative risk can also be used and would be more suitable in such circumstances.

4 Hierarchy of evidence and investigating causation

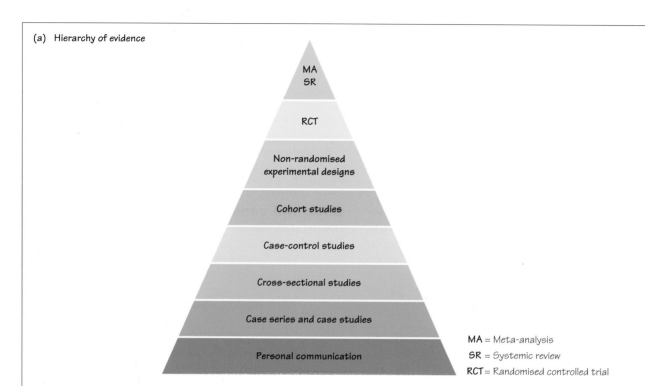

(a) Hierarchy of evidence

MA
SR

RCT

Non-randomised experimental designs

Cohort studies

Case-control studies

Cross-sectional studies

Case series and case studies

Personal communication

MA = Meta-analysis
SR = Systemic review
RCT = Randomised controlled trial

(b) Applying the Bradford Hill criteria to the evidence linking smoking and lung cancer

Bradford Hill criterion	Evidence of link between smoking and lung cancer
Strength of association	The relationship between smoking cigarettes and lung cancer is very strong
Dose-response relationship	The more cigarettes you smoke, the more likely you are to develop lung cancer
Temporality	Lung cancer takes around 20 years to develop: lung cancer prevalence only started to increase approximately 20 years after smoking prevalence increased in the same population
Consistency	The above relationships have been established in numerous studies in many different countries and populations
Biological plausibility	Cigarettes produce many substances that have been demonstrated to be carcinogens, but it is worth noting that none had been identified when the original epidemiological studies demonstrating the above links were undertaken
Reversibility	The risk of developing lung cancer reduces over time in those who have stopped smoking

Public Health and Epidemiology at a Glance, First Edition. Margaret Somerville, K. Kumaran, Rob Anderson.

Hierarchy of evidence

In public health, as in clinical medicine, we are concerned about using evidence to support our decisions and plans. Evidence can come from many sources and we find some sources and evidence more trustworthy than others. We may prefer to accept evidence or information because it comes from someone we trust, such as a senior colleague, an acknowledged expert or a family member rather than from a website, a newspaper or a commercial company interested in selling us their product. We may also recognise that some evidence is intrinsically more likely to be a reliable guide to action than others. For example, a large, well-conducted randomised controlled trial (RCT) testing a new drug against current treatment is more likely to convince us of the efficacy or otherwise of the new drug than an anecdotal report from one patient that they improved after taking it. In other words, we want to base our decisions, if possible, on evidence that is as unbiased and least subject to confounding or chance findings (see Chapter 5) as possible.

The hierarchy of evidence (Figure 4a) reflects this relative weight or value given to the different research methods and study designs. This forms an integral part of evidence-based practice particularly in making recommendations.

There are two main types of epidemiological studies:
• **Observational studies**, where the investigator observes natural occurrence. Examples include case-control, cohort and cross-sectional studies.
• **Experimental studies**, where the investigator intervenes actively. Examples include randomised controlled and non-randomised trials.

In general, experimental studies are given greater credence than observational studies, which in turn have greater weight than case reports.

The greatest weight is given to meta-analyses and systematic reviews of randomised controlled trials (see Chapter 10). Experimental study designs follow next in the hierarchy – a randomised trial is less subject to confounding than non-randomised trials (see Chapter 9). Observational studies follow next (see Chapter 8). The other weaker study designs are useful for generating hypotheses rather than establishing association or causation.

Some issues to consider:
• Weaker study designs provide useful information, especially where it is unethical to perform randomised trials. For example, the link between smoking and lung cancer was identified by observational studies.
• A well conducted observational study may provide better information than a poorly conducted RCT.
• Although the focus of this hierarchy is essentially on quantitative studies, it is important to use an appropriate study design to answer the question being asked (e.g. it is not ideal to use RCTs to determine the prevalence of a disease). Sometimes it may not be appropriate to use quantitative study designs at all and one would need qualitative studies to answer certain questions (e.g. what are the barriers to the uptake of primary care services). Qualitative studies complement quantitative studies and contributes to evidence-based practice by addressing questions which are relevant to making the best decisions for patients.

Establishing a causal relationship

An association between an exposure or risk factor and an outcome or disease does not imply that the risk factor causes the disease. Three possible factors (see Chapter 6) are important in considering whether a causal association really exists:
• Is the association due to a chance occurrence?
• Is it due to a flaw in the methodology (**bias**)?
• Is it due to some other factor linked to both exposure and outcome (**confounding**)?

Austin Bradford Hill, a British epidemiologist, detailed an approach for assessing evidence of causation. Although it has tended to be used as a checklist, it is important to remember that this was not his intention when he published his paper in 1965. He never used the term 'criteria' and stated that these points were not always necessary nor sufficient for causation. Although some of the points are of lesser value than others, they offer a systematic approach to critically appraise the evidence for causation.
• **Strength of association**: the stronger or greater the association, the more likely there is a causal relationship; this is usually indicated by large odds or risk ratios.
• A **dose–response relationship**: the higher the exposure to the risk factor, the greater is the incidence of disease.
• **Temporality**: the risk factor should precede the disease, and if there is an expected time period between exposure and outcome, the outcome must occur after that period has lapsed.
• **Consistency**: the same association is demonstrated repeatedly from multiple studies in different populations at different times by different investigators.
• **Biological plausibility**: a biomedical reason or factor that fits in with the known pathology of the disease adds weight to a causal relationship. However, this may be limited by current knowledge and should not be used to rule out a causal relationship completely.
• **Reversibility**: a reduction or withdrawal of the risk factor should result in a reduction or reversal of the outcome.

Figure 4b illustrates the application of these 'criteria' to the evidence linking smoking and lung cancer.

Bias, confounding and chance in epidemiological studies

(a) Observer bias leading to inaccurate results

Let us consider a study looking at smoking and lung cancer where an investigator assesses lung cancer using x-rays. Let us assume the true distribution is:

	Outcome	No outcome
Exposed	200	800
Unexposed	100	900

Risk in exposed = 200/1000 = 20%

Risk in unexposed = 100/1000 = 10%

Relative risk = 20%/10% = 2

Let us assume there were 5% borderline x-rays in both sets. If there were observer bias, and the investigator classified borderline x-rays in smokers as having lung cancer and similar x-rays in the non-smoker group as being normal, the table would look like:

	Outcome	No outcome
Exposed	250	750
Unexposed	50	950

Risk in exposed = 250/1000 = 25%

Risk in unexposed = 50/1000 = 5%

Relative risk = 25%/5% = 5

Thus even a 5% misclassification can potentially yield substantially misleading results

(b) Systematic and random error

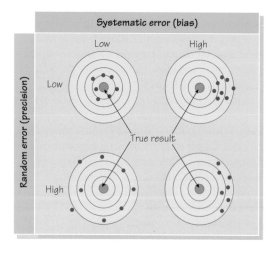

(c) A confounder is a variable that affects both exposure and outcome and therefore alters the relationship between them

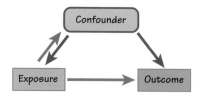

(d) P value and 95% confidence interval

A study looked at the effect of a new treatment drug A on curing an infection in comparison to the existing treatment drug B. Drug A cured 60% while drug B cured 40%.

The difference was 20% (95% CI 15-25) with a p value of 0.01.

These results suggest that drug A cured about 20% more in this study but at a population level, we are 95% confident that the difference in efficacy between the drugs is between 15 and 25%. Another way of expressing this would be to say that if we repeated the study 100 times in the same target population, we would expect to find a difference of between 15% and 25% on 95 of the occasions.

The p value suggests that, if there were really no effect, we would expect to find a result of this magnitude or greater only once in a hundred times.

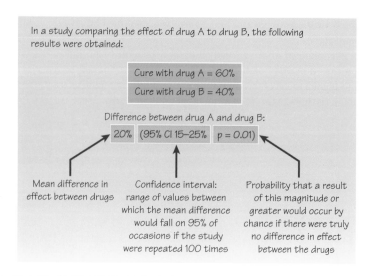

Public Health and Epidemiology at a Glance, First Edition. Margaret Somerville, K. Kumaran, Rob Anderson.

Evidence-based practice involves the critical appraisal of studies to assess their possible contribution to clinical or public health practice. When appraising studies, there are three main issues that need to be considered for their impact on the results:
• Bias
• Confounding
• Chance

The statistical analysis only reports how likely it is that the results have occurred by chance; it is important to recognise that a study can only be used to inform practice if it is well designed, so that the results are credible. If a study is not credible, then the results are of no value.

Bias

Bias is a systematic error or flaw in the methodology of the study which affects the results. There are two main types that we are likely to come across – selection bias and information bias.
• **Selection bias** is a flaw in the way subjects are selected for the study. Selection bias can occur when subjects selected are not representative of the population about which conclusions need to be drawn.
• **Information (or measurement) bias** can arise from errors in measuring exposure or outcome appropriately and can take several forms which may be relevant in different studies and settings.

In this chapter we consider mainly observer and recall bias; publication bias is considered in Chapter 10.
• **Observer bias** occurs when a researcher measuring the outcome has knowledge of the subject's exposure to a risk factor or intervention, and this knowledge affects how they assess outcomes. In borderline cases he/she might be more likely to classify exposed subjects as having the outcome and unexposed subjects as not having the outcome (Figure 5a).
• **Recall bias** occurs when a subject with the outcome is more likely to remember an exposure or other events than a subject without the outcome of interest.

In any study, there will be some element of random error. The smaller the random error, the more precise the study. Random error will tend to misclassify equally between the groups, unlike bias where there is a systematic misclassification in favour of one group (Figure 5b).

Confounding

Confounding is essentially an alternative explanation for the results. It occurs when a particular factor is associated with both the exposure and the outcome (Figure 5c). It can occur whether the exposure is truly a factor which affects the outcome or not. For example, if a study found out that physical activity reduced the incidence of coronary heart disease (CHD), then it could be that the physically inactive people were all older people. Both physical activity and age can have an influence on CHD incidence. However, consider another example where those who regularly drink more than 4 units of alcohol a day are found to have an increased risk of lung cancer. It may be that those who drink more also tend to smoke more and are therefore at greater risk of lung cancer. Here only smoking has an influence on lung cancer and not alcohol. In both of these examples, age and smoking are the confounders.

Confounding is an issue only if the confounder is unequally distributed between the two groups under comparison. For example, age is a confounder only if the physically inactive people were all older than the physically active group.

Confounding can be accounted for in the design stage of a study. For example, randomisation accounts for confounding by making the two groups under comparison as similar as possible by distributing the confounders equally between them. Another option is to adjust for confounders in the statistical analysis. For example, the relationship between physical activity and CHD could be examined in different age groups to see if the results are consistent. Another way of adjusting is by using regression methods (not discussed in this book).

Chance

Chance, or uncertainty in estimates, is mostly determined by sample size – the larger the sample, the greater the chance that the sample estimate of the population mean is closer to the true population mean. The impact of chance on the results of a study are usually expressed as **P values** and **confidence intervals**. In any epidemiological study, the starting point is to assume that there is no difference between the two groups being tested (i.e. the null hypothesis). If any difference is observed, then it is important to determine whether this observed difference could be due to chance or whether it is a real difference.

The magnitude of the P values helps to look at chance. The P value is the probability that an effect at least as great as that observed in the study could have occurred by chance alone, assuming there is no true relationship between exposure (risk factor or treatment) and outcome (disease or cure). The value for statistical significance is conventionally set at $P = 0.05$ (or less); it means that the probability that the effects observed could be due to chance alone is 1 in 20 (or less) if there were really no relationship between exposure and outcome measures. Obviously, the smaller the P value, the less likely the results are due to chance alone. However, 1 in 20 is an arbitrary figure adopted by the scientific community to indicate statistical significance. If we do 20 statistical tests in any study, there is a likelihood that one of those analyses will yield a P value of 0.05 or less, i.e. indicating statistical significance when there may in fact be no difference.

Confidence intervals, on the other hand, provide a measure of the robustness of the results. They provide an estimate or range within which the true answer will lie at a population level. It is important to remember that we can only be sure of the exact effect on our sample, although in reality we need to find out what is likely to be the effect at population level. The confidence intervals provide a range within which we can assume that the true value will lie at a population level. In practice, we tend to use 95% confidence levels, which provides us with a range within which we are 95% confident the true value lies. An alternative way to think about it is to assume that if we repeat the same study 100 times, the results would lie within the estimated confidence intervals 95 times (Figure 5d).

Confidence intervals are influenced by sample size. A small sample will usually yield wider intervals whereas a large sample will yield narrower intervals.

6 Standardisation

(a)

Age band	Numbers of Deaths			Populations				Age-specific death rates per 100,000 population		
	Town A	Town B	England & Wales	Town A	Town B	England & Wales		Town A	Town B	England & Wales
0–4	0	0	89	15443	6578	3324713		0	0	2.68
5–14	1	1	182	33096	14053	6683125		3.02	7.12	2.72
15–34	7	1	1213	74055	28625	14155299		9.45	3.49	8.57
35–64	138	90	32284	93305	44919	19588150		147.90	200.36	164.81
65–74	214	110	41735	21460	13539	4489813		997.20	812.47	929.55
75+	319	249	62254	18467	15699	3769060		1727.41	1586.09	1651.71
All ages	679	451	137757	255826	123413	52010160	Crude death rates	265.41	365.44	264.86

(b) Calculating the DASR

Age band	Expected numbers	
	Town A	Town B
0–4	0	0
5–14	202	476
15–34	1338	494
35–64	28971	39247
65–74	44772	36478
75+	65107	59781
Total	140390	136476
DASR	269.9	262.4

(c) Calculating the SMR

Age band	Expected numbers	
	Town A	Town B
0–4	0	0
5–14	1	0
15–34	6	3
35–64	154	74
65–74	199	126
75+	305	259
Total	665	462
SMR	101.9	97.5

Public Health and Epidemiology at a Glance, First Edition. Margaret Somerville, K. Kumaran, Rob Anderson.

Standardisation is often carried out to remove the effect of a particular characteristic in a group, in order to make valid comparisons between populations. The commonest characteristic adjusted for by standardisation is age, as illustrated by the example in this chapter, but other characteristics can also be adjusted for in this way, such as gender and socio-economic status. Standardisation is therefore a technique for adjusting for common known confounders in populations (see Chapter 5).

Why do we need to standardise data?

Disease measures such as death rates, prevalence or incidence vary with age for certain diseases. Most commonly in developed countries, incidence, prevalence and mortality for diseases such as cancer and heart disease increase with increasing age. Other diseases, such as some infections, occur more commonly at other ages.

When conducting an epidemiological investigation, we often want to compare disease measures in different populations, but if these populations have different age structures, then any differences we may see may simply be due to the effect of age. In epidemiological terms, age is a confounding factor (see Chapter 5). Standardisation is the technique that allows us to remove the effect of age when comparing disease measures between populations.

Types of standardisation

• **Direct standardisation:** the age-specific rates in the population of interest are applied to the proportion of people in each age band in a specified reference population. This method produces a **directly age-standardised rate (DASR).**

• **Indirect standardisation:** the observed mortality/morbidity pattern in a population is compared with what would have been expected if the age-specific rates had been the same as in a specified reference population. This method produces a standardised ratio (e.g. SMR, standardised mortality ratio or standardised morbidity ratio). By definition, the SMR for the reference population is 100. Areas, or population groups, with SMRs below 100 have a lower mortality/morbidity than the reference population and those with an SMR of above 100 have a higher mortality/morbidity.

• **Standard populations:** A national population structure is often used as the reference population, such as that of England and Wales, but standard populations have also been constructed for international comparisons, such as the European and World populations. Both DASRs and SMRs can be calculated using any population as the reference population.

Applications

Standardisation is most commonly done for age and sex, but can also be applied to other population characteristics or confounding factors, such as ethnicity or socio-economic status.

Example

Figure 6a shows the number of deaths from cancer in Town A, Town B and England and Wales in 1 year. As the purpose of this example is to demonstrate the technique of standardisation, we have used only six broad age bands; normally, 5-year age bands are used, from 0–4 to 85 and over. Also shown are the numbers of people and the age-specific death rates for each age band. Note that the crude all-ages death rates for Town A and Town B are very different, and that the two areas have different age structures, but that the age-specific rates are generally similar.

The DASR is calculated by multiplying each age-specific rate in Town A and Town B by the number in each age band for England and Wales. For example, the age-specific rate at age 35–64 for Town B is 164.81 per 100 000; multiplying it by the number in that age band for England and Wales gives us 39 247, which is the number of cancer deaths we would expect to see in England and Wales in the 35–64 age group if the Town B death rate for that group applied across the whole population . Summing the numbers across the age bands and dividing by the total population for England and Wales gives us the DASR, which is multiplied by 100 000 to give us a rate per 100 000 population, as shown in Figure 6b. Note that the rates for Town A and Town B are now very similar.

The SMR is calculated according to following formula:

$$\frac{\text{observed deaths/events in area}}{\text{expected deaths/events in area}} \times 100$$

The expected deaths are calculated by multiplying the age-specific rates for England and Wales by the population in each age band in Town A or Town B, as shown in Figure 6c. Again, Town A and Town B have very similar SMRs.

We can therefore conclude that the difference between the crude death rates in Town A and Town B is due to the differing age structures of the two populations. As both SMRs are also similar to the reference value of 100, we can also conclude that Town A and Town B have similar mortality to that of the reference (national) population. While DASRs can be compared with each other, SMRs cannot as they are comparisons with the reference population. While SMRs for Town A and Town B are similar to the national benchmark, they give no indication of whether cancer is a common or rare cause of death. If we are interested in investigating whether people in Town B are more at risk of developing cancer than people in Town A, perhaps due to local environmental exposures, the standardised rates and ratios are useful in removing the effects of age, but the actual numbers of people dying of cancer are more relevant if we are interested in planning cancer services.

7 Ecological and cross-sectional studies

(a) Correlation between neonatal mortality (per 1000), 1911–15 and coronary heart disease mortality (SMRs), 1968–78 among areas within England and Wales

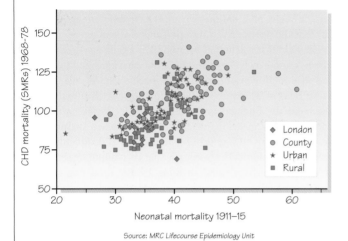

Source: MRC Lifecourse Epidemiology Unit

(b) Correlation between average life expectancy and GDP per person across countries

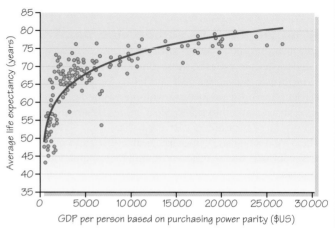

Source: From Lynch, J.W. et al., BMJ 2000;3320:1200–1204, accessed at bmj.com. ©200 BMJ Publishing Group Ltd

(c) Ecological fallacy

A classic example of ecological fallacy is the study on suicides by Emile Durkheim, a French sociologist. In his study on suicides, he discovered that rates of suicide were higher in predominantly Protestant areas in comparison with areas that were predominantly Catholic. He suggested that the rates were lower in the Catholic areas because of their greater social cohesion. However, an analysis at individual level undertaken suggested that Catholics living in Protestant areas had a higher rate of suicide compared with those Catholics living in mainly Catholic areas. Although there was still some suggestion that rates were slightly higher among Protestants at individual level also, the magnitude was far lower than it appeared to be at ecological level. It was suggested that Catholics living in predominantly Protestant areas were more socially isolated and therefore more likely to commit suicide than those living in Catholic areas. This study illustrated that a relationship that appeared to be true at the group level may not be true at an individual level.

Another example is a study in the US where states with the more recent immigrants were also found to have the highest prevalence of English literacy. Did this therefore imply that the new immigrants had better English literacy than the locally born population? In reality, from individual-level studies, the immigrant population had lower English literacy than the population born in the US. The immigrants tended to move to areas where the locally born population had higher literacy rates creating the ecological fallacy.

Source: Robinson W S 1950. Ecological Correlations and the Behavior of Individuals, American Sociological Review 15: 351–57

(d) An example of aggregation bias (exposure on x-axis and outcome on y-axis) where the group level data shows opposite findings to the individual level data

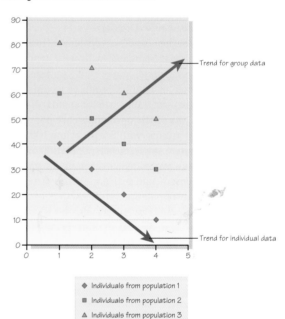

Public Health and Epidemiology at a Glance, First Edition. Margaret Somerville, K. Kumaran, Rob Anderson.
20 © 2012 John Wiley & Sons, Ltd. Published 2012 by John Wiley & Sons, Ltd.

Ecological studies

Most observational studies measure data at individual level. In an ecological study the unit of observation is at population or community (ecological) level. The disease or outcome and the exposure of interest are measured in a number of populations and their relationship is examined.

A common use of ecological studies is to look at geographical correlations. Figure 7a illustrates an example where coronary heart disease mortality correlates with infant mortality rates 60 years previously. This finding led to the hypothesis that impaired fetal development may lead to coronary heart disease and its risk factors in later life. Figure 7b shows the relationship between gross domestic product (GDP) and life expectancy at country level. Ecological studies may be used more where the key outcome of interest, such as equity of access, or an explanatory variable, such as GDP, can be measured better at an area or community level. Although ecological studies are useful for generating hypotheses, findings should be confirmed in more rigorous studies on individuals.

As in any other study, ecological studies are subject to **confounding** and **bias**. If the group level data come from very different populations – e.g. in terms of age, risk factor prevalence or ethnicity – then comparisons between them are difficult, as information on the confounders may be confined to the average population level.

Information bias is also a particular issue. Data collection may vary significantly between populations or countries, making it uncertain whether comparisons are valid. For example, if we use data from death certificates to compare death rates from coronary heart disease across countries, variation in the quality of death certification and completeness of reporting may account for any differences seen rather than variation in coronary heart disease prevalence, treatment or severity.

Ecological fallacy

There is a specific issue that we need to consider in ecological studies. Associations that appear true at a population level need not necessarily be true at an individual level. See Figure 7c for two examples of ecological fallacy.

A related or particular form of ecological bias is **aggregation bias** (a form of information bias): aggregated data may show an opposite effect to what is happening at individual level. An example is illustrated in Figure 7d. In the figure, where individuals from three different populations are assessed (with exposure along the x-axis and outcome along the y-axis), we can see there is a negative relationship at individual level between the exposure and outcome. However when these data are aggregated by population, it appears as though there is a positive relationship.

Time trends

Many diseases show fluctuations in incidence with time, and analysis of time trends may provide important information if such fluctuations correlate with other changes in the community. It may be easier to do this at population level. For example, the fluctuations in the incidence of coronary heart disease in the UK during the 20th century, which have been associated with changes in the prevalence of known risk factors for coronary heart disease, is discussed in Chapter 14.

Time trends are also of use in assessing the impact of vaccination programmes (see Chapter 26) and screening programmes. However, confounding can occur, just as in other studies, and it is important to be aware of other changes during that time period that may account for the findings.

In spite of their limitations, ecological and time trend studies are valuable because:
• The data is often abstracted from published statistics and the study may hence be quick and cheap to perform.
• Some exposures that occur at group level can be measured easily, e.g. air pollution, income, socio-economic indicators.

Cross-sectional studies

Cross-sectional studies are usually descriptive studies which may show an association between exposure and outcome, although an analytical element can be built into them.

Cross-sectional studies consist of a single examination of a population without any follow-up, i.e. data are collected at one point in time. They provide a 'snapshot' of a population and can measure attitudes, behaviours, health conditions (past and present) or risk factors (past and present), and can be repeated to measure change in a population. To conduct cross-sectional studies, we first need to define a **sampling frame**, i.e. a list of all those within a target population who can be selected as subjects. For example, the electoral roll or GP practice lists within a district can form the sampling frame. A simple random sample of subjects can be selected by a computer-generated list of random numbers from the sampling frame. If there is a need for particular subgroups (e.g. specific age groups), then the study population can be divided into subgroups (strata) and a sample can be selected from each subgroup.

Cross-sectional studies can be:
• **Descriptive:** measuring one parameter, e.g. prevalence of diabetes in adults over the age of 40.
• **Analytical:** measuring outcome and exposure, e.g. measuring prevalence of obesity in the same population as the prevalence of diabetes.

Although they cannot be used to measure incidence and are subject to bias and confounding as with any study, the specific issue of concern with cross-sectional studies is that of **temporality**; i.e. it is impossible to be certain whether an outcome developed before or after the exposure occurred. In the above example, it would be difficult to ascertain whether diabetes developed after individuals became obese or whether the individuals with diabetes tended to become obese after diagnosis.

The national census is a good example of a cross-sectional study of an entire population and provides a great deal of information on, for example, people's age, lifestyles, and living and working conditions. In the UK, a census is conducted every 10 years, providing denominator data for population studies and examining changes and trends over time.

8 Case-control and cohort studies

(a) Basic design of case-control studies

The investigator chooses the proportion of cases to controls depending on the required sample size; the most efficient study design is a 1:1 ratio.
In general, ratios of over 4 controls to 1 case do not offer much additional benefit

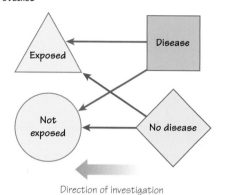

Direction of investigation

(b) Basic design of cohort studies

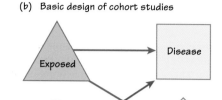

Direction of investigation

Box 8.1 Why we use odds ratio and not relative risk

Consider the example used in Chapter 3 to work out odds ratio where the proportion of cases to controls is 1:1

	Disease (lung cancer)	No disease (no lung cancer)	Total
Exposed (smoking)	90	30	120
Unexposed (no smoking)	10	70	80
Total	100	100	

Odds ratio of exposure in cases to controls = 21

If we were to work out relative risk:

Risk in exposed/Risk in unexposed = 90/120 / 10/80 = 6

Let us now change the proportion of cases to controls to 1:2. The table will now look like the following

	Disease (lung cancer)	No disease (no lung cancer)	Total
Exposed (smoking)	90	60	150
Unexposed (no smoking)	10	140	150
Total	100	200	

Odds ratio = 90/10 / 60/140 = 21
– i.e. same as previous value

Relative risk = 90/150 / 10/150 = 9
– quite different to the previous value!

Box 8.2 Comparing case-control and cohort studies

	Case-control studies	Cohort studies
Rare outcomes	Useful	Not useful
Rare exposures	Not useful	Useful
Multiple exposures	Useful	Can be used but difficult
Multiple outcomes	Not useful	Useful
Temporal relationship between exposure and outcome	Not clear	Usually clear
Measurement of incidence	No	Yes
Follow-up	Not usually an issue	Validity affected by poor follow-up
Emerging diseases	Useful in generating hypothesis	Less useful initially but useful to confirm hypotheses generated
Conducting a study	Usually faster and cheaper	Can be expensive and time consuming

Public Health and Epidemiology at a Glance, First Edition. Margaret Somerville, K. Kumaran, Rob Anderson.

Case-control and cohort studies are the most common epidemiological study designs used to examine an association between a risk factor (exposure) and disease (outcome). Chapter 4 gives an overview of investigating causation.

Basic design of case-control and cohort studies

In case-control studies, the outcome has already occurred at the time of investigation. Data on exposure to a potential risk factor is collected, usually from records or by administration of questionnaires.

Figure 8a illustrates the basic design of a case-control study. In a case-control study, we start off by recruiting a group of people who already have the disease of interest (i.e. the cases). We then use a group of people drawn from the same population who do not have the disease of interest (i.e. the controls). The cases and the controls are then compared for the prevalence of the risk factor of interest.

In cohort studies, in contrast, the outcome of interest has not occurred at the start of the investigation. People with and without the exposure of interest are followed up to examine the proportion in each group who go on to develop the outcome of interest. Occasionally in cohort studies, data on exposure in the past is collected, usually from documented records. The outcome may or may not have occurred at the time of the study in such instances. Figure 8b illustrates the basic design of a cohort study.

The cases and controls can almost always only be compared by using odds and odds ratios. Remember that as the investigator chooses the number of cases and controls, we cannot calculate risk (of developing disease) and measures of relative risk. Altering the proportion of controls to cases (keeping distribution of the exposure in the controls constant) will not change the odds ratio, but it will change the relative risk or risk ratio (see Box 8.1 for an example). Therefore the only statistical measure we can use in case-control studies is the odds ratio, comparing the likelihood of exposure in cases to controls.

In cohort studies, we can compare the risk of disease in the exposed and unexposed groups and calculate risks and risk ratios, and rate and rate ratios. We can also calculate odds ratios if necessary.

See Box 8.2 for a comparison of case-control and cohort studies. An example of using case-control and cohort studies to investigate an outbreak of food poisoning is given in the Appendix. See Chapter 3 for calculation of odds, odds ratios and measures of risk.

Key issues in case-control studies

• **Selection bias:** it is essential to ensure that the controls are drawn from the same population as the cases. The exposure to risk factors and confounders of the controls should be representative of the population at risk of developing disease. The cases and controls need to be as similar as possible except for the outcome.

• **Information bias:** it is likely that someone who has a disease will be more likely to remember an exposure compared to someone who does not have the disease (**recall bias**). It is difficult to eliminate this bias but it can be minimised by asking about a number of exposures in the same manner, so that the participants do not know what the exposure of interest is. There is also the possibility that the investigator may be more likely to look for potential exposure if aware of the outcome in a participant (**observer bias**); this can be minimised by the investigator not knowing the outcome and by collecting data on exposure from cases and controls in exactly the same manner.

• **Reverse causality:** As the outcome of interest has already occurred, it is difficult to know whether the exposure preceded or followed the outcome. This issue cannot be resolved definitively in case-control studies and will require other study designs to confirm findings.

Key issues in cohort studies

• **Follow-up:** it is essential that follow-up is as complete as possible for all participants. If there are any differences in follow-up, the differences and the possible reasons need to be explored. Where it is not explicit, assume that there are always likely to be differences between those followed up and those lost to follow-up.

• **Measurement bias:** can be minimised by collecting data on exposure and outcomes in the two groups as objectively as possible in the same manner.

Matching

Sometimes in case-control studies, cases are 'matched' to controls in terms of age and sex. This is usually performed to control for potential confounding factors (confounding is discussed in Chapter 5). It is, however, important to be wary of 'over-matching' which can occur when cases and controls are matched for factors that are not confounders but may be related to the exposure itself. When cases are matched individually with controls, it is important to keep in mind that a **matched pair analysis** is undertaken. It is always possible to adjust for potential confounders in the analysis as long as the confounder is known and the relevant information has been collected.

Nested case-control study

Occasionally, during a cohort study, when cases of disease occur, these cases can then be compared with controls to examine other possible risk factors. This design whereby cases are selected from within a cohort study is called a **nested** case-control study. This design is useful as it is often more efficient as cases and controls are drawn from the same cohort. It reduces information bias as the data has usually been collected at baseline.

9 Trials (experimental studies)

(a) Design of a trial

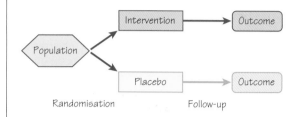

Randomisation   Follow-up

Box 9.1 Features of randomised controlled trials

Random allocation – distributes confounders (known and unknown) equally between the 2 groups

Blinding – ideally both investigators and participants should be unaware of the allocated treatment group - minimises bias (both observer and recall)

Follow-up –important as those lost to follow-up may differ from those who remain in trial. If losses are significant, the characteristics of those lost to follow up should be compared with those who remain at the end of a trial

Intention to treat analysis – groups analysed on the basis of original allocation - important because it maintains the balance in confounding, minimises bias and gives an estimate of effectiveness in real world settings

(b) Rationale for analysis by intention to treat

Randomisation generates two groups of people with similar proportions of mild (green) and severe (red) disease. One group is allocated to receive intervention and the other to receive placebo. During the course of the trial, some people in the intervention group do not get the treatment, while some in the placebo group do receive the active intervention. It may be that those with more severe disease in the placebo group will get the intervention while those in the intervention group who do not get treated have milder disease

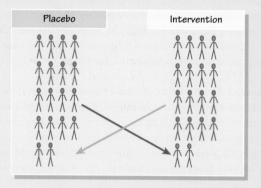

Analysing the groups by what they received may therefore be biased as the balance of mild and severe disease (and other confounders) produced by randomisation may have been altered

In real life, people do not take the treatment or always complete the course. Intention to treat analysis takes into account all of the above issues

(c) Calculating the Number Needed to Treat (NNT)

Let us consider antivirals for seasonal influenza in healthy people. If 40% become symptom-free after 5 days without antivirals and 60% become symptom-free after 5 days with antivirals, then the absolute risk reduction with antiviral use is 60-40 = 20%

Therefore the NNT is 100/20 = 5 i.e. we would need to treat 5 people with antivirals to achieve one additional cure from influenza after 5 days. We can also look at this pictorially –

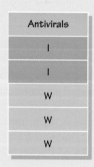 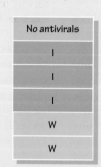

Antivirals
I
I
W
W
W

No antivirals
I
I
I
W
W

I = ill
W = well (after 5 days)

As shown above, for four of the five people treated, treatment would not make any difference to the outcome: only one person has recovered with treatment who would otherwise have remained ill without it

For calculating the number needed to harm (NNH), if 10% of those treated with antivirals developed diarrhoea (as opposed to none for the untreated group), the absolute risk difference would be 10-0 = 10%. This would result in a NNH of 100/10 = 10 i.e. for every 10 people treated with antivirals, one of them would suffer from drug induced diarrhoea

Public Health and Epidemiology at a Glance, First Edition. Margaret Somerville, K. Kumaran, Rob Anderson.

Trials are commonly used for evaluating the effectiveness of interventions, especially drug interventions. Most commonly, a new drug is compared to existing drugs or a placebo. The trials can be categorised as randomised or non-randomised depending on the method of allocating people to receiving either the interventional drug or placebo/existing drug.

In a randomised trial, the allocation of participants into either group is **random**, i.e. every participant who enters the study has an equal chance of receiving either the intervention or placebo. In non-randomised trials, the process of allocation is not random and may be predictable.

Trials (whether randomised or non-randomised) are essentially similar to cohort studies (see Chapter 8). The key difference is that participants are allocated to either an intervention group or a placebo group by the investigators. Figure 9a illustrates this situation, where the participants are randomly allocated to an intervention group and a control group. The groups are then followed up to assess the development of the desired outcome in each group. A variation of this design is a **cross-over trial**, where each group gets both treatment and control interventions. A period of 'wash-out' is needed whereby any residual effects of the treatments are eliminated, before each group is allocated to the other arm of the trial. The groups are then followed up for assessment of the outcome.

Key features of a good trial
Randomisation
Randomisation helps to distribute both known and unknown confounders equally between the intervention and control groups (see Figure 9b). If the groups are similar to each other in all aspects apart from the actual intervention itself, we can be more sure that any difference in outcome is due to the intervention and not due to other causes. Remember that there may still be differences between the groups, especially in small samples, and it is necessary to compare the characteristics of the two groups. **Concealment of allocation** refers to the process of protecting the randomisation so that the treatment to be allocated is not known to either the participants or the investigators before the patient enters the study.

Blinding
Blinding refers to the process where the treatment actually received is unknown to either some or all of the investigators, participants, assessors and analysts. Although traditionally terms such as **single blind** and **double blind** have been used to describe whether either one or both of the participants or investigators is blind to the treatment received, the terms are not helpful and it is better to specify whether the investigator or participants or both are blinded.

Blinding helps to reduce the possibility of information bias (such as observer or recall bias).

Follow-up
Having final outcomes measured for all or a high proportion of those allocated to treatment or control is essential, as for any study type. If follow-up rates are poor, it is important to compare the characteristics between those followed up and those lost to follow up. If there are no data, assume that those lost to follow up are different and therefore bias may be introduced.

Intention-to-treat analysis
This technique is used to deal with changes in protocol (where participants can take a treatment other than the one they were allocated) or those who drop out of the study. In this method, participants must be analysed on the basis of the group they are originally allocated to, even if they do not end up taking the treatment they were allocated. Allowing people to move or cross over between groups may make the groups less comparable and therefore disturb the balance in confounding achieved by the process of randomisation. The movement may also introduce bias, as those who move may be different in a way which affects the treatment effect. Finally, analysing people on original allocation will usually provide a better measure of its effectiveness in real world settings.

Measures of effect in randomised trials
All the measures of effect discussed in Chapter 3 can be used in randomised controlled trials (RCTs). An additional measure that is commonly used is the NNT (number needed to treat).

Number needed to treat and number needed to harm
The NNT is the inverse of the absolute risk difference (or 100 divided by the absolute risk difference if expressed as a percentage). The NNT is a useful measure which provides an indication of the effort required to achieve one additional cure (see Figure 9c). It provides a single number to consider the balance between benefits, costs and harm when the main outcome of interest can be defined as a binary event or health state. It is particularly used in drug intervention trials as it provides a single measure of effectiveness relative to the amount of treatment that needs to be provided. The number needed to harm (NNH) is similar, except that it looks at adverse effects rather than effectiveness. See Figure 9c for an example.

RCTs, when well performed, are the best possible research design for establishing an intervention's effectiveness as we can be very confident that any difference in outcome between the two groups is due to the intervention.

(a) A Forest plot is a common format for presenting the results of a systematic review, whether or not a meta-analysis has been undertaken. The results of each study included in the review are plotted either side of a vertical axis, with the horizontal axis indicating whether the result favours the treatment of interest or the comparator, which can be another active treatment or a placebo. If a meta-analysis has not been undertaken, then no diamond representing the pooled results from the individual studies appears on the Forest plot.

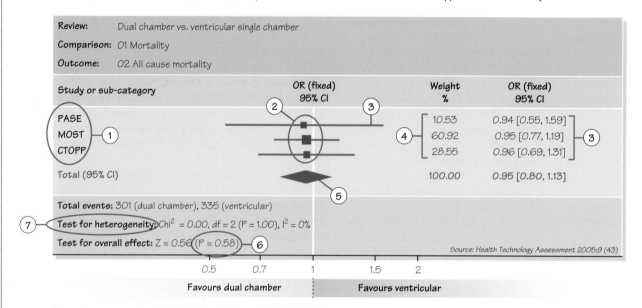

1 Names of trials

2 Individual trial results (usually Odds Ratios): the size of the square indicates the relative size of the study

3 The 95% confidence limits around the individual trial results

4 The weight each individual trial contributes to the overall pooled result; the weight roughly reflects the size of the study

5 Pooled result (missing if meta-analysis not undertaken): the points of the diamond indicate the 95% confidence limits

6 Significance of pooled result

7 Test for heterogeneity: p<0.05 indicates significant heterogeneity between studies is present

(b) Funnel plot – a measure of study size is plotted against its result, with small studies providing the wide base and big studies the narrow tip of a (roughly) inverted funnel shape. Because of sampling uncertainty (or chance) small studies show wider variation in their results than do bigger studies, but are expected to be distributed evenly around the pooled effect size. If publication bias is present, then small studies with negative results are likely to be missing (open circles on diagram), making the funnel plot asymmetrical.

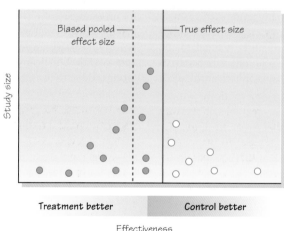

Public Health and Epidemiology at a Glance, First Edition. Margaret Somerville, K. Kumaran, Rob Anderson.

Systematic review

A systematic review attempts to identify, appraise and synthesise all the empirical evidence that meets pre-specified eligibility criteria to answer a given research question. Researchers conducting systematic reviews use explicit methods aimed at minimising bias, in order to produce more reliable findings that can be used to inform decision making (*Cochrane Handbook for Systematic Reviews of Interventions*).

A systematic review asks a clear, focused question and describes how the authors identified, appraised and synthesised the studies relevant to that question, minimising biases in the collation processes. Others should be able to reproduce the review. Systematic reviews are seen as the mainstay of evidence-based practice because there are often several, and sometimes many, effectiveness studies relevant to any given clinical or public health practice question. They do not have to be exhaustive, but should provide a search strategy and clear inclusion and exclusion criteria to account for the studies they have considered. For example, a review may only include randomised controlled trials (RCTs) or only studies published in the last 10 years. A systematic review can include any type of study; the approach is not confined to RCTs, but the quality and relevance of the studies should be appraised. Finally, a systematic review provides a synthesis of the included studies, which may be a quantitative pooling of the results by meta-analysis or a narrative synthesis or a combination of both.

The results of a systematic review are usually summarised in a forest plot, where the individual study results are plotted on a vertical axis (Figure 10a, items 1–3). Such a plot may not be possible where different studies use diverse outcome measures.

Publication bias

An explicit, reproducible search strategy and clear inclusion and exclusion criteria cannot fully compensate for publication bias. It is well recognised now that studies reporting 'positive outcomes' (e.g. that a new drug is better at lowering blood pressure than a placebo) are more likely to be published than those reporting 'negative' or inconclusive outcomes, particularly if the studies concerned are small. A **funnel plot** can help to assess whether a systematic review is affected by publication bias (Figure 10b). To reduce the chance of publication bias, authors can try to find relevant unpublished studies by

• searching registers of trials or of research in progress (e.g. the National Research Register in the UK)
• interviewing experts in the field to identify relevant researchers and unpublished studies.

Meta-analysis

Meta-analysis is a statistical technique for **quantitatively** pooling the results of individual studies. Studies that are pooled in this way may come from a systematic review, but do not have to. The results are usually shown in a Forest plot (Figure 10a, items 4–7). Studies should only be combined in this way if they are sufficiently similar; if they are not, then pooling the results does not yield a meaningful summary result. Heterogeneity is identified statistically (Figure 10a, item 7).

Heterogeneity can result from
• chance

• clinical differences between studies, such as different doses or duration of treatment
• different outcomes
• different populations
• methodological differences such as analytical methods, blinding or randomisation techniques.

If heterogeneity is present, then it should be explored. It may be more appropriate to analyse subsets of studies, e.g. those using the same outcome measures or methodologies, to remove the heterogeneity. Studies are probably best not combined if heterogeneity remains after such exploration and particularly if it cannot be explained.

The Cochrane Collaboration

The Cochrane Collaboration was launched in 1993 and is now an international network of centres and researchers with the aim of 'facilitating and coordinating the preparation and maintenance of systematic reviews of randomised controlled trials of health care'. It provides guidance on the conduct and reporting of systematic reviews and its many reviews are available online.

Systematic reviews of public health interventions

Systematic reviews are as highly valued for evaluating public health interventions and programmes as for assessing clinical treatments, but they present particular challenges. First, public health interventions may be provided by non-clinicians and outside health care settings, and so research about them may not be in medical journals or not published as research articles. Research about the effectiveness and cost-effectiveness of public health programmes is therefore often harder to find. Public health interventions are often multi-faceted, tailored to their context, and may target whole communities. As a result, they are not only hard to define, but usually also difficult to evaluate using high-quality study designs. Systematic reviews of the effectiveness of public health programmes therefore often yield no or few RCTs. Wider heterogeneity of study designs and outcome measures is more common, usually with considerable heterogeneity of results, so meta-analyses of the effectiveness of public health programmes are relatively rare. Despite these observations on the difficulties of systematically reviewing the effectiveness of public health interventions and programmes, RCTs and other rigorous study designs are as highly desirable in this field as in health care. Just as in health care, what appears to be a plausible intervention to improve health may not prove to be the case when subjected to rigorous evaluation. Increasingly, it has been demonstrated that public health interventions and programmes can be evaluated using RCT methodology.

Questions to ask when appraising a systematic review and meta-analysis

• Did the review ask a clear and focused question?
• Is a clear and detailed search strategy described?
• Could important and relevant studies have been missed?
• Were the criteria for including studies stated and appropriate?
• Were the included studies appraised for quality and relevance?
• Were the results similar across studies?
• How were the results synthesised and presented?

11 Diagnostic tests

(a) Sensitivity, specificity, predictive values and likelihood ratios

The graph shows the distribution of test results for the normal population (in blue) and the diseased or abnormal population (in red). The same information can also be presented in a 2x2 table. The definitions use the same annotation.

		Disease		
		Positive	Negative	Totals
Test	Positive	a	b	a + b
	Negative	c	d	c + d
	Totals	a + c	b + d	a + b + c + d

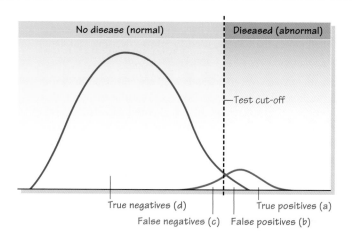

Sensitivity is the proportion of people **with** the condition correctly identified by the test: .... $\dfrac{a}{a+c}$

Specificity is the proportion of people **without** the condition correctly identified by the test: .... $\dfrac{d}{b+d}$

Positive predictive value is the proportion of those **with a positive test** who truly have the condition: .... $\dfrac{a}{a+b}$

Negative predictive value is the proportion of those **with a negative test** who truly do not have the condition: .... $\dfrac{d}{c+d}$

Positive likelihood ratio is the likelihood of a positive test in those with the condition divided by the likelihood of a positive test in those without the condition .... $\dfrac{a/a+c}{b/b+c}$ or $\dfrac{\text{Sensitivity}}{1-\text{Specificity}}$

Negative likelihood ratio is the likelihood of a negative test in those with the condition divided by the likelihood of a negative test in those without the condition .... $\dfrac{c/a+c}{d/b+d}$ or $\dfrac{1-\text{Sensitivity}}{\text{Specificity}}$

Prevalence of the condition: $\dfrac{a+c}{a+b+c+d}$

(b)

In both scenarios, test sensitivity and specificity are the same, at 99% and 99.9% respectively, but in scenario A (prevalence 0.1%) the positive predictive value is 49.7%, while in scenario B (prevalence 10%) it is 99%. The likelihood ratios are the same in each scenario: LR pos 990 and LR neg 0.01

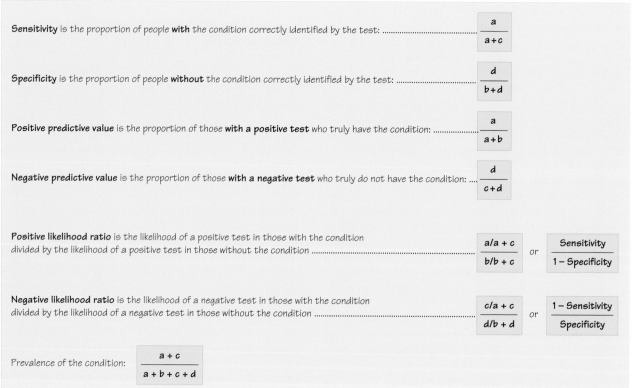

Scenario A Prevalence 0.1%		Disease		
		Positive	Negative	Totals
Test	Positive	99	100	199
	Negative	1	99 800	99 801
	Totals	100	99 900	100 000

Scenario A Prevalence 10%		Disease		
		Positive	Negative	Totals
Test	Positive	9900	90	9990
	Negative	100	89 910	90 010
	Totals	10 000	90 000	100 000

Public Health and Epidemiology at a Glance, First Edition. Margaret Somerville, K. Kumaran, Rob Anderson.

Clinicians carry out investigations on patients in order to make a diagnosis. A diagnostic test can range from a physical examination, such as measuring blood pressure, to a blood test, such as haemoglobin levels, or performing a radiological examination. Data obtained from these tests can be either continuous, i.e. the result can take any value within certain limits, or non-continuous, e.g. normal or abnormal. Continuous data can be plotted as a frequency distribution (Figure 11a). The ability to label test results as coming from those with and without the condition assumes that there is a 'gold standard' which can truly identify those with and without the condition being tested for. Comparing the diagnostic test with the gold standard allows the test results to be separated into two distributions, for those who do or do not have the condition of interest. As no diagnostic test can perfectly separate these two groups, the two distributions always overlap and a threshold value has to be set, above which people are classified as having the condition being tested for, and below which they are classified as normal. The overlapping distributions of results from the two groups, however, means that there will always be some people **with** the condition whose test result is below the threshold (false negatives) and some people **without** the condition whose result is above the threshold (false positives)

Sensitivity, specificity, predictive values and likelihood ratios

A good diagnostic test should ideally be able to identify as many of those with the condition as possible and exclude from further investigation and treatment as many of those without the condition as possible. The former characteristic of a test is its **sensitivity** and the latter its **specificity** (see definitions in Figure 11a).

Sensitivity and specificity are useful in deciding whether a test will miss a significant proportion of people with the condition or fail to exclude people without the condition. They are not particularly helpful when it comes to interpreting a test result for an individual. **Predictive values** give us the probability that a positive test result means that the patient does have the condition, or that a negative result means they do not have the condition.

To be useful in practice, a diagnostic test should also alter our initial estimate of how likely it is that an individual has the condition in question. The initial probability of an individual having the condition is simply given by the prevalence of the condition in the population. **Likelihood ratios (LR)** enable us to alter that pre-test probability depending on the test result. If a test is positive, a high positive LR (LR pos >10) will increase the post-test probability of having the condition substantially, while a low positive LR (<0.1) will reduce the post-test probability substantially. If a test is negative, a high negative LR (LR neg >10) will increase the post-test probability of having the condition and a lower negative LR (<0.1) will decrease the post-test probability of having the condition sub-

stantially. Values for LRs of around 1 are unhelpful as they do not alter our pre-test probability.

Effect of prevalence on predictive values and likelihood ratios

Diagnostic tests are performed on a wide variety of populations, from unselected populations, such as those invited for screening, to highly selected patient groups attending specialist services. These populations vary in terms of their prevalence of the condition being tested for. While the sensitivity and specificity of the test remain unchanged, predictive values alter with the underlying prevalence in the population being tested (Figure 11b). In contrast, likelihood ratios do not change as disease prevalence alters.

Screening tests

In the special case of screening a population for a specific condition, a very sensitive initial test is required, so that very few people with the disease are missed, i.e. there are very few false negatives. Ideally, it should also be very specific, so that very few people without the disease are identified for further investigation and treatment, i.e. there are very few false positives (see Chapter 27). In practice, high sensitivity is usually preferred to high specificity, so that few cases are missed, but false positives are identified that need excluding from treatment by further testing.

In other circumstances, a highly specific test may be preferred to ensure that few false positives are identified and treated, but at the expense of missing some cases as false negatives.

Checklist for appraising studies of diagnostic tests

Did clinicians face diagnostic uncertainty?

Was the test performed on the right spectrum of patients, i.e. did the patients represent the usual presentations of the condition in question, along with commonly confused diagnoses?

Was there a blind comparison with an independent gold standard?

The 'gold standard' or reference standard is usually a biopsy, autopsy or other confirmation that the individual does have the condition under investigation. Those performing the gold standard test should not know the results of the initial test.

Did the results of the test being evaluated influence the decision to perform the gold standard test?

The gold standard test should be performed on all those who were given the initial test, regardless of that test result. If the gold standard test involves risky invasive procedures, then those with a negative test may be followed up long-term to check that they do not develop the condition at a later date.

(a) The pre-requisites for health as set out in the Ottawa Charter for Health Promotion (WHO 1986)

The fundamental conditions and resources for health are:

- Peace
- Shelter
- Education
- Food
- Income
- A stable eco-system
- Sustainable resources
- Social justice and equity

Improvement in health requires a secure foundation in these basic requirements

(b) Geographical distribution of the prevalence of limiting long-term illness in England and Wales in 2001

The map shows the proportion of people who answered "yes" to the following question in the 2001 UK census:

Do you have any long-term illness, health problem or disability which limits your daily activities or the work you can do?

The proportions responding "yes" vary from 10.9% to 30.7% across England and Wales

People with a limiting long-term illness as a percentage of all people

- 20.94 – 30.77
- 18.30 – 20.98
- 16.80 – 18.09
- 14.73 – 16.79
- 10.93 – 14.72

Source: www.erpho.org.uk/viewResource.aspx?id=14346

(c) Pyramid illustrating the spectrum of disease severity

Dead

Admitted to hospital

Illness managed in primary health care

Symptoms, but not seeking help from health services

Asymptomatic, but found to have disease on testing

Healthy

Definition of health

The World Health Organization (WHO 1948) has defined health as

> a state of complete physical, mental and social well-being and not merely the absence of disease or infirmity.

This definition has not been amended since the WHO Constitution was adopted in 1946, and was re-affirmed by the Declaration of Alma Ata (1978). Few could disagree with it as an aspiration, but it does pose problems of whether everyone, at an individual and population level, can realistically achieve such a state. The WHO has gone on to discuss how health for all can be achieved, through the Ottawa Charter for Health Promotion (WHO 1986):

> To achieve a state of complete physical, mental and social well-being, an individual or group must be able to identify and to realise aspirations, to satisfy needs and to change or cope with the environment. Health is, therefore, seen as a resource for everyday life, not the objective for living.

The Charter also set out what it considered to be the prerequisites for health (Figure 12a).

The chapters in this section of the book cover the sources of data for describing and analysing health and its determinants and describe the health impacts of some of the main determinants. Many other factors also influence health; this book is not comprehensive in its coverage of information that may be relevant in assessing the health of a population. Health promotion is covered in Chapters 29 and 30.

Illness

Concepts and beliefs about illness vary widely within and between cultures and communities. Views of health professionals on the causation of illness, as well as on the best way to manage it, may also differ from those of the lay population and in some cases from those of other health professionals.

Whether or not a person seeks help from health professionals depends on many factors. Such factors include the nature and severity of the symptoms (people are more likely to seek help for symptoms that start abruptly or are perceived as worrying) and the disruption the symptoms cause to everyday activities such as work or childcare.

From a public health perspective, understanding health beliefs and why and when people consult health services is essential to plan and develop health services and preventive programmes that people will use and find effective. It is particularly important to understand why some population groups, referred to as 'hard to reach', do not use services and to consider ways in which they can be encouraged to do so. Some ethnic minorities, travelling communities and young single men can all be considered hard to reach for some services.

Disability, impairment and handicap

These three terms are useful in describing the actual physical problem caused by an illness (**disability**), the function that cannot be carried out as a result of that problem (**impairment**) and the resulting impact of that lack of function on the person's life and everyday activities (**handicap**). Similar disabilities and impairments have very variable impacts on different individuals. For example,

most people may be able to cope with the loss of a finger, but to a professional musician it may mean the loss of their livelihood.

Measuring health and illness

Many of what are termed measures of health are actually measures of illness. Routinely available health data include numbers and causes of death, diagnosed cases of specific diseases such as cancer or communicable diseases, prescribed drugs and contacts with health services, e.g. consultations and hospital admissions.

General health is usually measured subjectively by asking people whether they are well or not. There are a number of standard questionnaire-based tools that can be used to measure general health in surveys, clinical trials or other research studies. Commonly used measures include the SF36 (Short Form 36), the GHQ (General Health Questionnaire), the EQ5D and the NHP (Nottingham Health Profile). The topic of measuring health and quality of life, particularly for use in economic evaluations, is covered in Chapter 32.

Illness can also be measured subjectively, by asking patients to rate their illness in terms of, for example, symptoms, symptom severity or ability to perform everyday activities. For instance, the UK census contains a question on whether people have any long-standing illness which limits their activities (Figure 12b). There are many tools available for use in specific diseases, e.g. Beck's Depression Scale and the St George's Respiratory Questionnaire.

Estimates of disease prevalence or incidence will inevitably depend on which methods of disease measurement have been used. For every person who dies of a disease, more are admitted to hospital with severe symptoms, far more are treated in primary care without the need for hospital admission, and many more again are symptomatic but do not seek help from health services. It is also possible that people may have a disease without becoming symptomatic: serological testing of a population for chickenpox or influenza, for example, will reveal those who have been infected but who have no history of a relevant symptomatic illness. This symptom pyramid or iceberg is shown in Figure 12c.

Example

Asthma is a common chronic disease characterised by variable wheeze and/or breathlessness, but it is not easily or succinctly defined, leading to difficulties in estimating prevalence. The following data demonstrate the difference in estimated prevalence, depending on the definition used:

Ever wheezed	33%
Wheezed in last 12 months	19%
Doctor-diagnosed asthma ever	21%

(Source: The Burden of Lung Disease: A Statistics Report from the British Thoracic Society, 2006)

In 2001, a combined variable of recent wheeze, asthma diagnosis ever, and treatment for asthma gave an overall prevalence of 8.1% in England. Prevalence of GP-treated asthma from primary care registers in 2004/05 was estimated at 5.8%, ranging from 3.2% to 7.4% across England (Source: Lung and Asthma Information Agency, 2006).

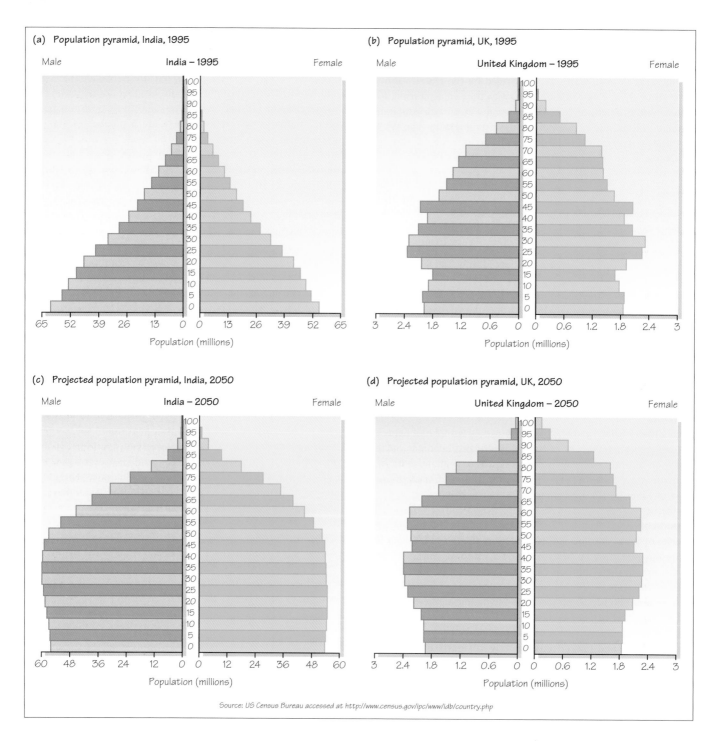

(a) Population pyramid, India, 1995

(b) Population pyramid, UK, 1995

(c) Projected population pyramid, India, 2050

(d) Projected population pyramid, UK, 2050

Source: US Census Bureau accessed at http://www.census.gov/ipc/www/idb/country.php

Public Health and Epidemiology at a Glance, First Edition. Margaret Somerville, K. Kumaran, Rob Anderson.

As public health involves the health of populations, it is important to be able to assess population health. Such an assessment is complex and involves the consideration of data at population level from a range of sources. They can be broadly divided into three types of data:

• Population descriptor data
• Health/illness data (Chapters 15 and 16)
• Lifestyle data (Chapter 17).

This section considers data that describes populations. The accurate assessment of population health requires an understanding of the numbers and characteristics of the people who are at potential risk of ill health. Data that are solely related to health or illness events cannot be interpreted without an understanding of the underlying population which provides denominator data.

A population census is one of the most important sources of population data and is carried out in many countries. It provides a periodic count of the number and characteristics of the people living in a defined geographical area. The census started in 1801 in the UK and is carried out every decade (it was not carried out in 1941 because of the Second World War). Data are collected on individuals and households. Information is collected on all individuals in a household and includes gender, date of birth, marital status, ethnic origin, country of birth, usual address, employment, education and self-reported health issues. Information collected on households includes postcode, number of rooms, type of dwelling and certain amenities.

Population pyramids and demographic transition

A population pyramid is a histogram of the age and gender distribution of a population. The age structure of a population changes as a country develops, its population becomes healthier and birth and death rates change. This change is referred to as the demographic transition and is closely related to the epidemiological transition described in Chapter 14, as the changing age structure reflects changes in disease patterns and their consequences as countries develop. Figures 13a and 13b show the population pyramids for India and the UK in 1995 while Figures 13c and 13d show the projected population pyramids for 2050. The shape of the population pyramids suggests that India is lagging behind the UK in terms of its demographic transition by about half a century.

The demographic transition model describes the changes that occur as a country or population moves through stages of development from a population with high fertility and mortality to one with low fertility and mortality. In the early stages of development, both birth and death rates are high with poor living conditions and health care provision. Infant and childhood mortality is high and infectious diseases are a major cause of death. Therefore the population grows relatively slowly. In the next stage, the birth rate continues to remain high while there is a fall in death rates due to improvements in living conditions and health care. Infections as a cause of death also begin to decline. This change results in a rapid growth in population. The third stage is characterised by a fall in birth rates while death rates remain low, usually the consequence of improved access to contraception, improved literacy of women, increasing urbanisation and the tendency to educate children, with a lower value placed on children's work. The final stage is characterised by a stable population with low birth and death rates. However more recently, a slight decline in population has been noted in certain countries in the developed Western world as a result of increasing life expectancy, very low birth rates and low death rates.

This model was developed based on the experiences of developed Western nations and may not be reflected in exactly the same manner in some developing economies. For example, the UK went through its demographic transition mainly between 1750 and 1950. In India the demographic transition has been relatively slow but steady, although occurring more rapidly than in the UK, while other countries are experiencing more rapid changes in population numbers and age structure.

A major limitation of the model is that it does not take into account the effect of migration. It also does not take into account epidemics, pandemics or wars which can kill large numbers of people including those in the young adult age group; this may not only affect the shape of the pyramid but also have an impact on the fertility rates.

A country which is in the early stages of development with a high birth and death rate has a population structure that is pyramid shaped. As it progresses through the stages of development with lower birth and death rates, it eventually becomes barrel shaped. A declining population can have an inverted pyramid shape.

The population pyramid can therefore be useful to understand the age and sex distribution of a population as well as birth and death rates. It also allows us to understand the number and proportion of those who would be considered economically dependent (under 16s and over 65s for most developed countries). Understanding the basic population structure forms a key component of appropriate service planning.

The UK has seen an increase in the proportion of over 65s and a decrease in the under 16s when comparing data over a 25-year period from 1984 and 2009. There has been a doubling of numbers in the 'oldest old' age group (over 85s) from 1% of the population to 2%. The ageing population has major implications for health and social care service planning and delivery in the future.

14 Epidemiological transition

(a) Top five causes of death in children under 5 years old in 2002

World	European region	African region
Pneumonia	Pneumonia	Malaria
Diarrhoeal disease	Low birth weight	Pneumonia
Low birth weight	Diarrhoeal disease	Diarrhoeal disease
Malaria	Injuries	HIV/AIDS
Measles	Meningitis	Measles

Data sourced from the WHO and UNICEF

(b) Mortality in Infants and children under 5 years old in 1990 and 2008

	Infant mortality rate (per 1000 live births)		Under five mortality rate (per 1000 live births)	
	1990	2008	1990	2008
Industrialised countries	8	5	10	6
Developing countries	68	49	99	72
Least developed countries	113	82	179	129
World	62	45	90	65

Data sourced from UNICEF

(c) Mortality from coronary heart disease and other causes (males aged 35 – 74 years), UK 1921-1994

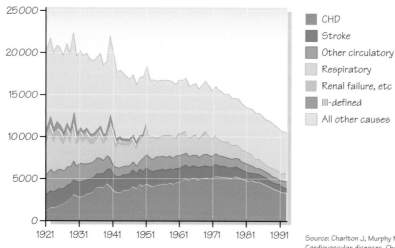

Legend:
- CHD
- Stroke
- Other circulatory
- Respiratory
- Renal failure, etc
- Ill-defined
- All other causes

Deaths per million population
(age standarised to European population)

Source: Charlton J, Murphy M, Khaw K-T, Ebrahim S, Davey Smith G. Cardiovascular diseases. Chapter 18 In: Eds: Charlton J, Murray M. *The Health of Adult Britain: 1841–1994.* Office of National Statistics. Decennial Supplement No. 13. The Stationery Office, London, 1997.

Public Health and Epidemiology at a Glance, First Edition. Margaret Somerville, K. Kumaran, Rob Anderson.

As countries progress through the stages of demographic transition, there is usually an accompanying epidemiological transition, as rates of certain diseases decline and others become more common. Infectious diseases as a major cause of mortality and morbidity decline while there is an increase in mortality and morbidity from chronic non-communicable diseases, which affect older age groups.

Figure 14a shows the top five causes of death in children under the age of 5 years across the world, the European region and African region. We can see that there are differences in the top causes of death reflecting differences in stages of transition: all five top causes in the African region are communicable diseases, while low birth weight and injuries appear in the European top five. The world top five reflects the African causes more than the European, because of the small numbers of deaths occurring in the European region compared to the African. The difference in infant and under-5 mortality across country groupings is seen in Figure 14b. While death rates are falling across all countries, the rates in developing and least developed countries are still many times higher than those in developed countries, reflecting the continuing high rates of infectious diseases in the former.

The general shift in the burden of mortality and morbidity from infectious diseases and malnutrition characteristic of underdevelopment to non-communicable diseases characteristic of development is referred to as the epidemiological transition. The process is complex as disease patterns alter as a result of demographic, socioeconomic and technological changes in a society.

As a country develops, there is a reduction in infant and under-5 mortality rates (infant mortality rate is considered to be a sensitive indicator of development), which impacts on the overall life expectancy of a population. As life expectancy increases, people live longer to ages where non-communicable chronic diseases such as heart disease and cancers become manifest.

Coronary heart disease (CHD) is a good case example. In England, the age-adjusted mortality rates from CHD in people aged 40–75 years increased more than fourfold between 1921 and 1945 (Figure 14c). This rise in mortality continued until the early 1970s. Subsequently a decline in CHD mortality in the UK began in 1973–74 and is still continuing. Initially mortality from CHD was higher in the upper socio-economic groups, but there was a gradual shift with time. The disease increased steadily in lower socio-economic groups while remaining relatively stable in the higher groups. By the 1950s CHD was higher in the lower socio-economic groups compared to the more affluent groups. Just as the rise was more marked initially in people from the upper socio-economic groups, so was the decline.

The changes in CHD patterns are consistent with demographic and epidemiological transitions that would be expected as a country progresses through stages of development. This pattern with CHD can also be seen in other parts of the world. Infectious and parasitic diseases as causes of death in developing countries are declining while CHD as a cause of death is increasing. The WHO predicted in 1996 that CHD will be the leading cause of death and disability worldwide by 2020. Countries and regions around the world tend to go through these epidemiological transition stages at differing times and speeds. For example, rates of CHD have increased rapidly in India recently. The increase in CHD has been attributed partly to a demographic transition as people are now living longer to an age where CHD develops. The increasing urbanisation of the population, changes in diet, lack of physical activity and increased presence of conventional risk factors are also contributory factors. This change has been accompanied by an epidemiological transition where there has been a decrease in infectious and parasitic diseases.

With the burden of disease now shifting to developing countries, population-wide efforts to control and reduce conventional risk factors across the life course are necessary to minimise the impact of CHD in the future.

Types of health data

	Routinely collected data	Specifically commissioned data collections
Mortality	Registration of deaths	
Morbidity	National health surveys e.g. Health Survey for England, Scottish Health Survey Disease Registers e.g. Cancer Registry Notifications of Infectious Diseases Primary care data on diagnoses of long-term conditions e.g. diabetes	Prevalence studies for specific diseases Enhanced surveillance systems (Chapter 25)
Health care activity	In-patient stays Outpatient consultations Prescribing Procedures e.g. hip replacements Investigations, e.g. X-rays, blood tests Contacts with health professionals e.g. community nurses, physiotherapists	Observational studies of the activities of specific services or staff groups
Determinants of health	Housing registers Water quality Unemployment figures Educational attainment Income Welfare benefits claimants Homeless household data Education participation (young people) Under-18 conception rate Low birthweight babies Breast-feeding initiation and prevalence at 6-8 weeks after birth	Local surveys on lifestyle risk factors

Public Health and Epidemiology at a Glance, First Edition. Margaret Somerville, K. Kumaran, Rob Anderson.

36 © 2012 John Wiley & Sons, Ltd. Published 2012 by John Wiley & Sons, Ltd.

Data sources

Information about the health of individuals is collected in various ways (see Figure 15). Contacts with health services, such as clinic consultations, hospital admissions, investigations and procedures, recording of cases of specific illnesses, such as cancer, and the certification of death all provide health information. Data from such sources are referred to as **routinely collected** or **administrative** data, and are used for a variety of purposes. Individual patient management, accounting and planning are usually the main reasons for such data collection. Because routine data are often not collected with an epidemiological purpose in mind, data quality may be an issue, due to incomplete records, lack of or inconsistent coding and misclassification.

Health information may also be collected through specific surveys. Survey data sources primarily provide counts of health events; to calculate rates of death or illness in a population, a denominator is required. National census surveys provide data on population numbers and many other characteristics (see Chapter 13). The quantity and availability of routine data sources in developed countries has increased enormously over recent years, with the development of appropriate information technology infrastructure, but variation between countries remains considerable.

In order to make comparisons between different populations, or over time, health events are often classified by the main underlying disease of the person experiencing them; the most widely used system is the International Classification of Diseases (ICD), now in its tenth revision.

Mortality

It is mandatory in most countries for every death to be registered. In the UK, a medical practitioner must issue a medical certificate of the cause of death, which records details of the person's age, sex, place of residence and occupation as well as immediate and contributing causes of death. Mortality data from this source is probably the most reliable health data available, in terms of completeness and accuracy, and provide a good indication of the nature of more serious health problems in a population. However, such data tell us little about long-term and non-fatal conditions, such as arthritis or psychiatric illness.

Mortality is most commonly expressed as crude death rates, standardised death rates or ratios (see Chapter 6) or age, sex and cause-specific death rates.

Morbidity

Estimates of rates of ill-health, or morbidity, in a population will vary according to the data source used. Those obtained from hospital or primary care records are likely to be lower and less reliable than those obtained by specific population-based surveys, particularly for conditions with a spectrum of mild to severe disease; those with mild disease may not consult health services. In the UK and other countries, there are regular population-based surveys of health, using clear objective definitions of disease. Such surveys also permit accurate collection of data on risk factors for illness, such as smoking and alcohol consumption. The Health Survey for England is conducted annually; core data are collected each time, with additional topics (such as cardiovascular disease or child health) being covered less frequently. Such surveys are essential to provide accurate information on incidence and prevalence of specific conditions.

For most conditions, routine records are more likely to provide disease prevalence than incidence data. Drug prescriptions for maintenance therapies for chronic diseases, such as diabetes or asthma, may be a good proxy for prevalence of doctor-diagnosed or more severe levels of chronic illness.

Disease registers exist for many diseases, covering different populations, and are of variable quality. The most comprehensive and high-quality registers require substantial resources to maintain them. Cancer registries now exist in many countries and provide high-quality information on the incidence, prevalence and survival for different cancers. Other registries record communicable diseases, and congenital and genetic conditions.

Health care activity

All health care systems have methods to capture activity, such as consultations, admissions, prescribing, surgical and other procedures, investigations and referrals. These systems have primarily been set up to manage individual cases and to ensure payment for services. Using such data for epidemiological purposes can be problematic, as it is often not clear what population is making use of the services. Case definitions and disease classification may also be inaccurate or unclear.

In hospital care, episodes of care tend to be recorded, rather than basing information on individual admissions. Primary care records provide information based on individuals; the Quality and Outcomes Framework in the UK is leading to better and more consistent health information which captures clinical quality as well as health service activity. As health systems develop their IT and communications systems, data quality is improving. Electronic patient records are becoming a reality in some countries, creating new opportunities for analysing linked service use and disease information.

Determinants of health

Information regarding the underlying determinants of health, such as environmental, socio-economic and educational factors, is often not available from routine health data sources. Providing a comprehensive description of the health of a population requires information from other sources, such as local government data on air or water quality, accidents, housing and income. Periodic national census, household and social surveys also provide important information relating to variations in key social indicators which are related to poor health or health care use.

16 Measuring population health status

(a) Comparison of summary measures of population health in a developed country (UK), a low mortality developing country (China) and a high mortality developing country (Afghanistan)

	UK	China	Afghanistan
Life expectancy at birth (years)[1]	80	74	42
Infant mortality per 1000 live births[1]	5	18	165
Probability of dying between the ages of 1 and 5 years per 1000 population[1]	6	21	257
Probability of dying between the ages of 15 and 60 per 1000 population[1]	78	113	479
Healthy Life Expectancy (years)[2]	72	66	36
Proportion of Years of Potential Life Lost (YPLL) by cause[3]:			
Communicable disease	7	20	77
Non-communicable disease	84	59	18
Injuries	9	21	5
Maternal mortality per 100,000[4]	8	45	1800

Source: World Health Statistics 2010 www.who.int 12008 data; 22007 data; 32004 data; 42005 data, using interagency estimates

(c) Attributable fraction (exposed) and attributable fraction (population)

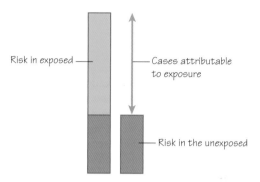

Attributable fraction (exposed)

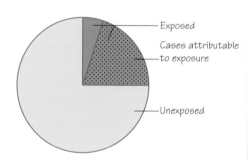

Attributable fraction (population)

(b) Diagrammatic illustration of perinatal, neonatal and infant mortality

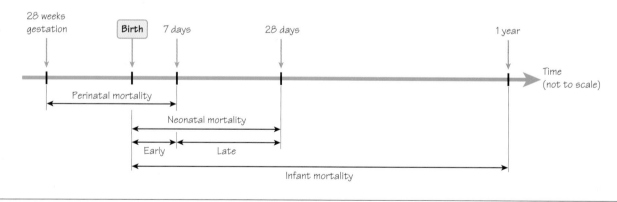

Assessing health status of a population

The health of a population can be described in general terms and in relation to specific conditions. A health status profile usually considers population-level mortality rates, age, sex and cause-specific mortality rates, the prevalence and incidence of specific diseases and the prevalence of specific risk factors such as smoking or alcohol consumption. It may be compiled from routinely collected data sources or through conducting specific surveys or studies (see Chapter 15).

Summary measures of population health

Two commonly used measures of a population's health are life expectancy at birth and infant mortality. Both are used to compare population health nationally and internationally (Figure 16a).

Life expectancy at birth is the average length of time that babies born today can expect to live if today's age and sex-specific mortality rates applied throughout their lifetime. It therefore provides a useful summary of current mortality rates in a population, and is a good indicator of that population's overall health. It cannot, however, be used to predict individual lifespans. As mortality rates are generally falling, babies born today are likely to live longer on average than today's mortality rates currently predict. Life expectancy is reduced more by deaths in infancy and childhood than by deaths at older ages.

Healthy life expectancy (HLE) combines measures of morbidity with mortality to give an average length of time that a person in a specified population can expect to live free of disease. It provides a better means of comparison for populations with high life expectancy due to low premature mortality from common fatal diseases such as heart disease and cancer, but high levels of illness due to diseases with low mortality rates such as depression and musculoskeletal conditions. **Disability-adjusted life years** (DALYs) provide a similar summary measure, which includes the years of potential life lost due to premature mortality and the years of productive life lost due to disability (see Chapter 33) (www.who.int).

The **fertility rate** in a population is the number of live births per 1000 women of child-bearing age (usually taken as 15–44 years).

Infant mortality is a key measure reflecting the health of a population, particularly the health of pregnant women and the care given during childbirth, to newborn babies and to infants. The infant mortality rate is the number of deaths that occur in the first year of life in a specified population divided by the number of live births in that population. It is divided into several different periods (Figure 16b); deaths in each period are influenced by different factors. Perinatal mortality (stillbirths after 28 weeks' gestation plus deaths in the first 7 days after birth per 1000 live births plus stillbirths) are heavily influenced by maternal health, care during childbirth and factors leading to premature birth. Neonatal mor-

tality (deaths in the first 28 days after birth per 1000 live births) also reflects maternal health and care during childbirth as well as congenital conditions. Infant deaths after the neonatal period are most influenced by childhood conditions such as vaccine-preventable and diarrhoeal diseases, accidents and malnutrition. Infant mortality is generally very low in developed countries, where the main causes of death in this period are congenital conditions and accidents. In developing countries, in contrast, communicable diseases and malnutrition are the main causes of the higher mortality rates.

Years of potential life lost (YPLL) is an alternative method of summarising mortality rates, which takes account of the age at which death occurs. They are usually calculated as the years of potential life lost before age 75 years, so that deaths occurring at younger ages, such as those from accidents, influence the summary measure more than those occurring at older ages. For example, a death at age 20 years from a road traffic accident incurs 55 YPLL compared to a death at age 70 years from a heart attack, which incurs 5 YPLL.

Survival is usually used in relation to a specified disease, rather than as a measure of population health, and is therefore most useful in monitoring the success of particular treatment strategies. It can be calculated in several ways. The **crude survival rate,** directly calculated, is the number of people alive at the end of a specified period of time expressed as a proportion of those who were alive at the start of the period, or from diagnosis. **Corrected survival** distinguishes between those dying from the specific disease of interest and those dying of other causes. **Relative survival** compares the survival of a particular patient or population group to a group from the general population of similar age, sex and other characteristics.

The **attributable fraction (exposed)** is the proportion of disease in an exposed population that would be eliminated by removing a specific causal exposure (Figure 16c):

$$AF(exposed) = \frac{\text{risk in the exposed} - \text{risk in the unexposed}}{\text{risk in the exposed}}$$

The **attributable fraction (population)** is the proportion of a disease in the general population that is associated with a risk factor. It therefore takes the prevalence of the risk factor into account:

$$AF(population) = \frac{\text{risk in the population} - \text{risk in the unexposed}}{\text{risk in the population}}$$

These two measures are used to calculate the burden of disease attributable to specific risk factors in a population. They are also referred to as **attributable risk** and **population attributable risk**.

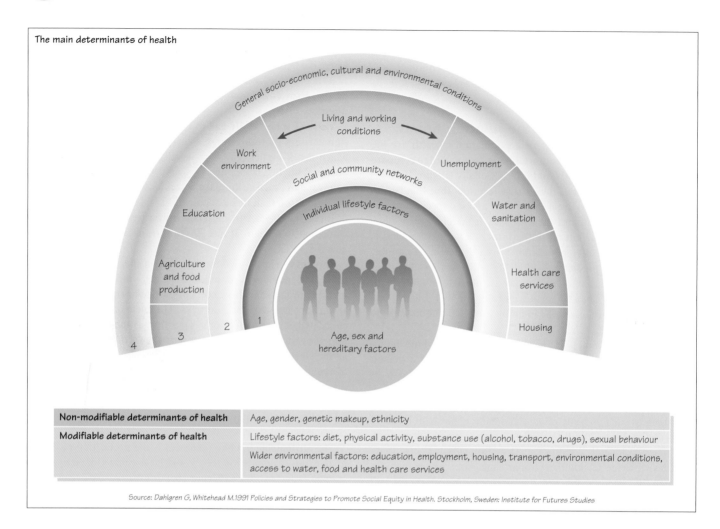

The main determinants of health

Non-modifiable determinants of health	Age, gender, genetic makeup, ethnicity
Modifiable determinants of health	Lifestyle factors: diet, physical activity, substance use (alcohol, tobacco, drugs), sexual behaviour
	Wider environmental factors: education, employment, housing, transport, environmental conditions, access to water, food and health care services

Source: Dahlgren G, Whitehead M.1991 Policies and Strategies to Promote Social Equity in Health. Stockholm, Sweden: Institute for Futures Studies

An individual's health is determined by a range of factors, some of which can be modified at an individual or wider environmental level. A useful framework for considering these influences is provided by the Dahlgren and Whitehead model (see Figure 17). The table lists examples of modifiable and non-modifiable factors. This chapter describes the influences of lifestyle risk factors on health, while the next two consider inequalities in health and the wider environment.

In affluent societies, diseases relating to obesity, tobacco smoking and alcohol consumption have replaced communicable diseases and malnutrition as major causes of premature mortality. The same patterns of disease related to lifestyle risk factors are emerging in developing countries as they get richer and adopt the lifestyles of more affluent countries.

The leading global risks for mortality in the world are high blood pressure (responsible for 13% of deaths globally), tobacco use (9%), high blood glucose (6%), physical inactivity (6%), and overweight and obesity (5%). These risks are responsible for raising the risk of chronic diseases such as heart disease, diabetes and cancers. They affect countries across all income groups: high, middle and low. The leading global risks for burden of disease as measured in disability-adjusted life years (DALYs) are underweight (6% of global DALYs) and unsafe sex (5%), followed by alcohol use (5%) and unsafe water, sanitation and hygiene (4%).

Eight risk factors (alcohol use, tobacco use, high blood pressure, high body mass index, high cholesterol, high blood glucose, low fruit and vegetable intake, and physical inactivity) account for 61% of cardiovascular deaths. Combined, these same risk factors account for over three-quarters of ischaemic heart disease, the leading cause of death worldwide. It is worth noting that over 84% of the total global burden of disease they cause occurs in low- and middle-income countries. Reducing exposure to these eight risk factors would increase global life expectancy by almost 5 years (Source: *WHO Global Health Risks 2009*).

The attributable fractions (AFs) quoted in the tables below are for the general population, not the populations exposed to the risk factor (see Chapter 16). The AF (population) takes the prevalence of the risk factor into account; the more prevalent the risk factor, the higher the proportion of disease in a population that can be attributed to it.

Public Health and Epidemiology at a Glance, First Edition. Margaret Somerville, K. Kumaran, Rob Anderson.

Table 17.1 Smoking-related diseases

Disease	Attributable fraction (% DALYs)
Lung cancer	71%
Ischaemic heart disease	10%
Respiratory disease	42%

Source: WHO Global Health Risks 2009, www.who.int.

Table 17.2 Population attributable fractions for selected diseases (% DALYs)

	Global	Developed countries
Direct harms		
Alcohol use disorders[a]	100	100
Liver cancer	25	28
Oesophageal cancer	29	36
Liver cirrhosis	32	49
Indirect harms		
Motor vehicle accidents	20	18
Homicide	24	32

[a]Alcohol use disorders are those conditions which by agreed definition are caused solely by alcohol, such as alcohol dependence, abuse, and toxicity and gastritis, neuropathy and cardiomyopathy due to alcohol.
Source: WHO Global Status Report on Alcohol 2004, www.who.int.

Table 17.3 Obesity attributable fractions of some conditions

Disease	Attributable burden of disease
Type II diabetes	90%
Hypertension	66%
Cancers (in non-smokers)	10%
Primary infertility in women	6%

Source: *Tackling Obesities: Future Choices Foresight Report 2007*, www.foresight.gov.uk.

Tobacco

Cigarette smoking became widespread amongst European men after the First World War, reaching a peak prevalence of 70–80% around 1950 in the UK and other Western countries, followed by a steady decline to around 25% of the adult male population in the early 21st century. For women, the peak prevalence of smoking occurred later and the decline has been slower.

Smoking-related diseases include lung, upper respiratory tract and upper gastro-intestinal cancers, ischaemic heart disease, stroke, peripheral vascular disease and chronic obstructive pulmonary disease (COPD). The proportion of specific diseases attributable to smoking tobacco is shown in Table 17.1. DALYs take account of both morbidity and mortality attributable to smoking (see Chapter 16); globally, 12% of male and 6% of female deaths are attributable to smoking.

Alcohol

Unlike tobacco smoking, alcohol consumption has been part of the culture of most societies for centuries. Globally, alcohol consumption is highest in European countries, but there is wide variation between countries and social groups within countries in the amount of alcohol consumed per capita, the form (as beer, wine or spirits) and the frequency, quantity and circumstances in which it is consumed. Such drinking patterns range from those who do not drink alcohol at all, through social drinkers, to binge and dependent drinkers. Alcohol consumption is very price-sensitive and fluctuates with levels of economic prosperity, taxation and price relative to average income.

Sensible drinking levels have been defined as up to 21 units of alcohol for men a week and up to 14 for women; a unit is defined as 10 ml pure alcohol.

Alcohol-related health harms can be classified as direct and indirect, with direct harms being sub-divided into acute and chronic. Table 17.2 gives the population alcohol-attributable fractions, as a percentage of all DALYs, for selected conditions, showing that the AFs generally increase in developed countries, where alcohol consumption is generally higher and other causes of the conditions are less prevalent.

Obesity

The prevalence of obesity (body mass index [BMI] >30 kg/m^2) and overweight (BMI >25 kg/m^2), has been increasing rapidly over the last 30 years in Europe in both adults and children. The causes of this increase are complex. Weight gain, at an individual physical level, results from an imbalance between energy intake and energy expenditure, but the reasons for excess intake over expenditure lie in the complex interplay of changes in eating habits, availability of cheap, energy rich foods, living and working patterns and levels of physical activity.

Table 17.3 shows the obesity AFs of selected conditions. In addition, overweight and obesity increases risk of ischaemic stroke, disability due to osteoarthritis in elderly people, obstructive sleep apnoea, impotence and infertility in men, and ischaemic heart disease.

(a) Measuring the environmental burden of disease

(i) Main diseases contributing to the environmental burden of disease

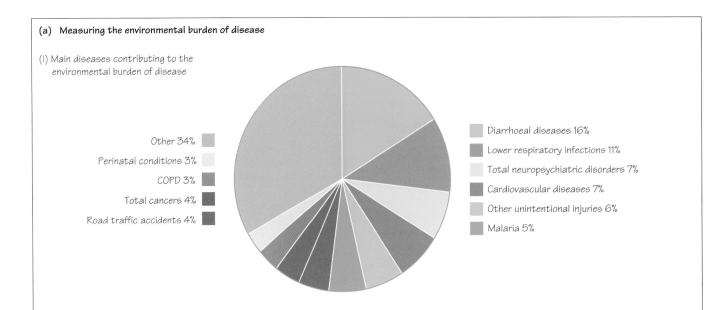

Other 34%
Perinatal conditions 3%
COPD 3%
Total cancers 4%
Road traffic accidents 4%

Diarrhoeal diseases 16%
Lower respiratory infections 11%
Total neuropsychiatric disorders 7%
Cardiovascular diseases 7%
Other unintentional injuries 6%
Malaria 5%

(ii) The diseases with the largest absolute burden attributable to modifiable environmental factors

Disease	Proportion of disease attributable to the environment	Modifiable environmental risk factors
Diarrhoea	94%	Unsafe drinking water, poor sanitation and hygiene
Lower respiratory conditions	20% in developed countries, up to 42% in developing countries	Indoor air pollution from household solid fuel use, second-hand tobacco smoke, outdoor air pollution
Malaria	42%	Policies and practices regarding land use, deforestation, water resource management, improved drainage, house design and siting of settlements

Source: Preventing disease through healthy environments WHO 2006 www.who.int

(b) Impact of human activity on the natural environment and some human health consequences

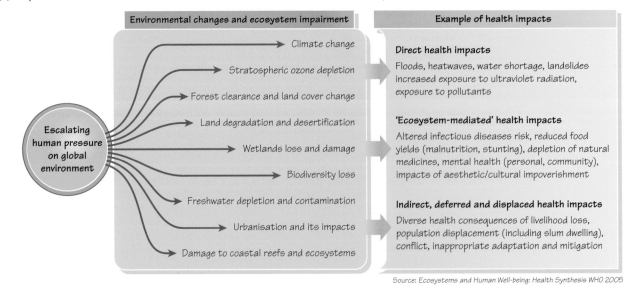

Environmental changes and ecosystem impairment	Example of health impacts

Escalating human pressure on global environment

Climate change
Stratospheric ozone depletion
Forest clearance and land cover change
Land degradation and desertification
Wetlands loss and damage
Biodiversity loss
Freshwater depletion and contamination
Urbanisation and its impacts
Damage to coastal reefs and ecosystems

Direct health impacts
Floods, heatwaves, water shortage, landslides increased exposure to ultraviolet radiation, exposure to pollutants

'Ecosystem-mediated' health impacts
Altered infectious diseases risk, reduced food yields (malnutrition, stunting), depletion of natural medicines, mental health (personal, community), impacts of aesthetic/cultural impoverishment

Indirect, deferred and displaced health impacts
Diverse health consequences of livelihood loss, population displacement (including slum dwelling), conflict, inappropriate adaptation and mitigation

Source: Ecosystems and Human Well-being: Health Synthesis WHO 2005

Public Health and Epidemiology at a Glance, First Edition. Margaret Somerville, K. Kumaran, Rob Anderson.

Many aspects of the natural environment can affect human health. In 2006, the World Health Organization (WHO) estimated the burden of disease from modifiable environmental factors and concluded that:

Globally, an estimated 24% of the disease burden (healthy life years lost) and an estimated 23% of all deaths (premature mortality) was attributable to environmental factors.

The burden in developing countries was proportionally greater than in developed countries (25% vs. 17%) and children were also more affected: among children aged 0–14 years, 36% of deaths were attributable to the environment (Figure 18a).

The conventional view of the natural environment, as described above, is the impact it has on human health, but people also have a major impact on the natural environment. By activities such as clearing forest, overfishing or the release of pollutants to the environment, humankind affects the quality of the water we drink and the air we breathe and risks the sustainable supply of healthy food. Given the choice, people prefer to live in a secure, predictable, attractive and diverse setting and may suffer ill health when such conditions deteriorate. Figure 18b sets out some of these consequences of human activity on the natural environment.

This chapter provides an overview of the interaction between the environment and human health. While thoughtful management and planning can minimise some of the more damaging impacts, events such as tsunamis or earthquakes are outside human control. The impact of such disasters is devastating and demands the rapid mobilisation of a range of agencies to address the immediate requirements of people who have lost homes, families and livelihoods and the longer-term needs of the physically injured and traumatised.

Environmental health

Environmental health comprises those aspects of human health, including quality of life, that are determined by physical, chemical, biological, social and psychosocial factors in the environment. It also refers to the theory and practice of assessing, correcting and preventing those factors in the environment that can potentially affect adversely the health of present and future generations (Environmental Health 2012 www.cieh.org)

In most countries there is now a substantial body of legislation aimed at protecting people from environmental hazards. Monitoring and ensuring compliance with such legislation is part of the public health function usually carried out by specialised environmental health practitioners. Air and water quality, waste management and disposal, food safety and noise levels are all aspects of the environment subject to regulation in this way. Ionising radiation, noise and risks arising through occupational exposure (for example to asbestos) are also regulated.

Air quality

Air pollution arising from burning fossil fuels is associated with respiratory and cardiovascular diseases. The London smog of 1952, a 4-day period during which levels of sulphur dioxide and particulates, or smoke, were 5–6 times higher than normal, is thought to have caused over 4000 deaths. This episode led to the establishment of standards for air quality in the UK, through the Clean Air Act, and UK levels of air pollution have diminished substantially as a result. Increasingly, road traffic contributes to air pollution in developed countries, as contributions from industrial and other sources diminish.

In many developing countries, the use of solid fuel on open cooking fires leads to substantial indoor air pollution and is a major cause of respiratory disease (Figure 18a).

Water quality

Water polluted by human and animal waste or toxic chemicals can pose a major threat to human health, and ensuring a safe drinking-water supply is a major public health objective. While such a supply is generally achieved in developed countries, for the rest of the world the need for effective water treatment is pressing; diarrhoeal diseases caused by water-borne infections account for around 1.4 million child deaths a year (Figure 18a). Major improvements in water quality can be achieved by preventing human waste contaminating the watercourses from which drinking-water is drawn. In the absence of a sewage treatment system, simple measures such as pit latrines, frequent hand-washing and safe storage of drinking-water can substantially reduce the occurrence of water-borne diseases. Nevertheless such systems cannot remove damaging contaminants from the water supply, and natural toxins, industrial wastes and agricultural run-off must still be managed and controlled if human health is to be maintained.

Malaria is a significant threat to health in many tropical areas. Poor land management and sanitation can result in areas of standing water in which malarial mosquitoes can breed. Drainage, use of insecticide-treated bed-nets and public education can combine to reduce the incidence of the disease.

Impact of climate change

Climate change is already happening; rising sea levels, reduction in suitable land for agriculture and buildings, food and water shortages and increased frequency of extreme weather events all impact on health. Warming of the ocean and atmosphere is changing patterns of land use, the availability of food and water supplies, the distribution of disease vectors and the frequency of extreme weather events such as floods and droughts. Such changes will interact to give new global patterns of human mortality and morbidity, and in many of the world's poorest countries there will be population migrations to more benign locations, creating a substantial strain on health services. Even if we stopped using fossil fuel today, warming would continue for some decades and thus it is vital that health services worldwide adopt policies that both adapt to a warmer planet and reduce (mitigate) the impacts of warming on human health.

19 Inequalities in health

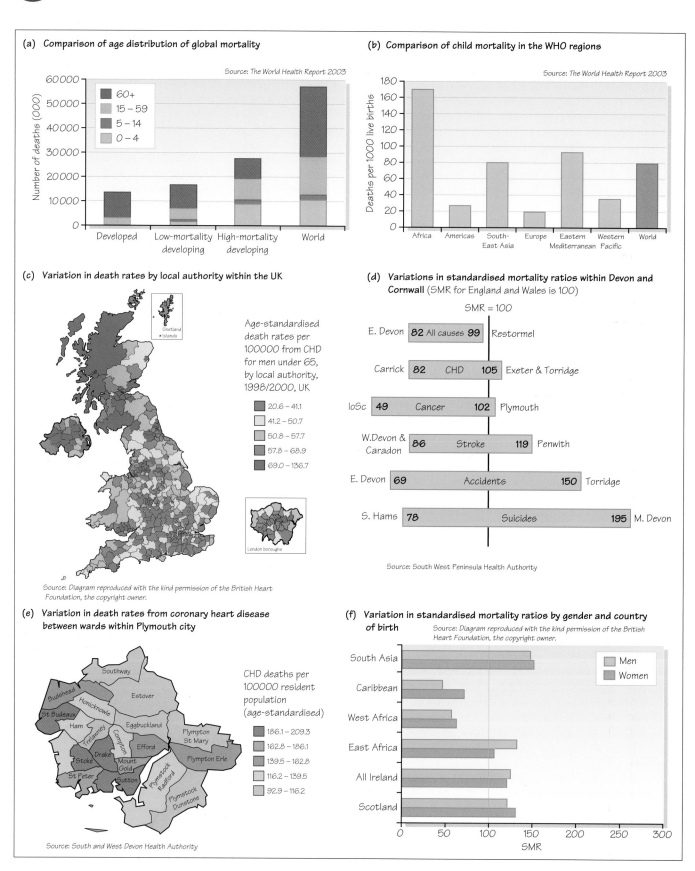

(a) Comparison of age distribution of global mortality

Source: The World Health Report 2003

Number of deaths (000)

60+
15 – 59
5 – 14
0 – 4

Developed | Low-mortality developing | High-mortality developing | World

(b) Comparison of child mortality in the WHO regions

Source: The World Health Report 2003

Deaths per 1000 live births

Africa | Americas | South-East Asia | Europe | Eastern Mediterranean | Western Pacific | World

(c) Variation in death rates by local authority within the UK

Shetland Islands

Age-standardised death rates per 100000 from CHD for men under 65, by local authority, 1998/2000, UK

20.6 – 41.1
41.2 – 50.7
50.8 – 57.7
57.8 – 68.9
69.0 – 136.7

London boroughs

Source: Diagram reproduced with the kind permission of the British Heart Foundation, the copyright owner.

(d) Variations in standardised mortality ratios within Devon and Cornwall (SMR for England and Wales is 100)

SMR = 100

E. Devon	82	All causes	99	Restormel
Carrick	82	CHD	105	Exeter & Torridge
IoSc	49	Cancer	102	Plymouth
W.Devon & Caradon	86	Stroke	119	Penwith
E. Devon	69	Accidents	150	Torridge
S. Hams	78	Suicides	195	M. Devon

Source: South West Peninsula Health Authority

(e) Variation in death rates from coronary heart disease between wards within Plymouth city

Southway
Budshead
Estover
Honicknowle
St Budeaux
Ham
Eggbuckland
Trelawney
Compton
Plympton St Mary
Efford
Stoke
Drake
Mount Gold
Plympton Erle
St Peter
Sutton
Plymstock Radford
Plymstock Dunstone

CHD deaths per 100000 resident population (age-standardised)

186.1 – 209.3
162.8 – 186.1
139.5 – 162.8
116.2 – 139.5
92.9 – 116.2

Source: South and West Devon Health Authority

(f) Variation in standardised mortality ratios by gender and country of birth

Source: Diagram reproduced with the kind permission of the British Heart Foundation, the copyright owner.

Men
Women

South Asia
Caribbean
West Africa
East Africa
All Ireland
Scotland

SMR

Public Health and Epidemiology at a Glance, First Edition. Margaret Somerville, K. Kumaran, Rob Anderson.

The problem of 'inequalities'

Health inequalities can be defined as differences in the health status of one group of people compared with another. These groups are commonly defined by age, sex, ethnicity, geography, social class, income and education.

Geographical inequalities

Inequalities in health are commonly demonstrated across geographical areas. Over the past 50 years, average life expectancy has increased globally by about 20 years – from 46.5 years in the 1950s to 65.2 years in 2002. However, this rise in life expectancy is not uniform across countries or continents. For example, the average life expectancy for a woman in a developed country is about 78 years compared to about 46 years for a man in sub-Saharan Africa.

Figure 19a illustrates differences in the age distribution of mortality patterns globally. For example, 60% of deaths in developed countries occur in the over 70s compared to just 30% in developing countries. Figure 19b shows the differences in child mortality in the six WHO regions. Of the 20 countries with the highest child mortality, 19 are in Africa (the other one is Afghanistan).

These inequalities exist not just between countries but also within countries. Figure 19c shows the variation in age-standardised death rates by local authority within the UK. These geographical variations are also seen at smaller levels: Figure 19d and 19e illustrate the variation in standardised mortality ratios (SMR) between local authority areas within Devon and Cornwall for selected causes (SMR for England and Wales is 100) and the variation in death rates due to coronary heart disease (CHD) at ward level within Plymouth city.

Other factors associated with inequalities

Factors such as age, gender and ethnic origin are also associated with differences in health status. Rates of CHD increase with age: Figure 19f shows variations in standardised mortality ratios from CHD by gender and country of origin. There is also evidence from other countries – for example, life expectancy at birth among indigenous Australians is lower in both men and women by over 15 years compared to all Australians.

Many of the factors responsible for inequalities in health are related to social and economic inequalities in society, between population groups and geographical areas. Deprivation indices (usually related to geographical area) and socio-economic status (usually related to occupation) are commonly used to highlight differences in health status between population groups.

Deprivation indices

Socio-economic status is usually, as the name suggests, a composite indicator based on information such as a person's occupation, employment status, educational attainment or income, and/or household and material characteristics such as home or car ownership. Measurements of socio-economic status are complex. Within the UK, the most commonly used indicators are the Townsend Score and the Index of Multiple Deprivation (IMD). Both of these scores can be used at small area level.

The **Townsend Score** is made up of four variables which include employment, car ownership, owner occupation and overcrowding. These variables are derived from the census: the higher the score, the greater the deprivation. Although this score is easy to calculate and correlates with measures of ill health, the data may be out of date as the census is only conducted every 10 years. It does not indicate the proportion of people in each area that are deprived and is usually a better measure of urban rather than rural deprivation (e.g., in a rural area car ownership may be a necessity).

The **IMD** is based on seven domains (Box 19.1). Each domain includes a number of indicators. Summary measures for these domains are aggregated to provide an overall measure of multiple deprivation and each area is allocated a score and rank. The higher the score, the greater is the degree of deprivation. Within the UK, separate indices have been developed for England, Wales, Scotland and Northern Ireland. Although conceptually similar, there are variations in the number of indicators used and the way in which they are defined between the four countries. Hence it is not possible to combine them together into a single UK index.

Since 2001, socioeconomic status has been based on the National Statistics Socioeconomic Classification (NS-SEC). This has replaced social class based on occupation (the former Registrar General's Social Class Classification, which had five groups). The NS-SEC was updated in 2010 (see Box 19.2) and is based on occupation; there are provisions to cover the whole of the adult population including those not in employment. There are eight groups, with the first one having two subdivisions.

Globally, inequalities in health are closely related to material deprivation where the burden of disease is often greatest in the poor. While absolute material poverty is relatively rare in a developed country such as the UK, there are still large inequalities in health between different groups which is related to income differentials between them. Chapter 20 discusses socioeconomic inequalities in more detail.

Box 19.1 Domains of the Index of Multiple Deprivation (IMD)

1 Crime
2 Education, skills and training
3 Employment
4 Health deprivation and disability
5 Barriers to housing and services
6 Income
7 Living environment

Box 19.2 NS-SEC classes (modified 2010)

1 Higher managerial, administrative and professional occupations
  1.1 Large employers and higher managerial and administrative occupations
  1.2 Higher professional occupations
2 Lower managerial, administrative and professional occupations
3 Intermediate occupations
4 Small employers and own account workers
5 Lower supervisory and technical occupations
6 Semi-routine occupations
7 Routine occupations
8 Never worked or long-term unemployed

(a) Comparison of mortality rates in men according to social class between 1930s and early 1990s

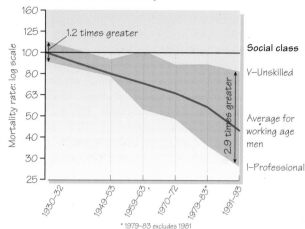

1.2 times greater

2.9 times greater

Social class

V–Unskilled

Average for working age men

I–Professional

* 1979–83 excludes 1981
England and Wales. Men of working age (varies according to year either aged 15 or 20 to age 64 or 65)
Source: Office for National Statistics, Decennial Supplements, analysis by DH Statistics Division

(b) Age standardised mortality rates by occupational groups in men aged 25–64, England and Wales, 2001–03

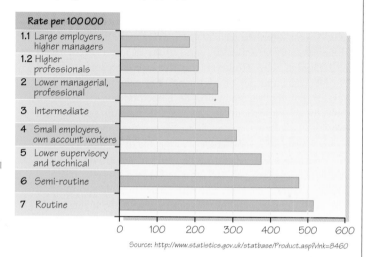

Rate per 100 000	
1.1	Large employers, higher managers
1.2	Higher professionals
2	Lower managerial, professional
3	Intermediate
4	Small employers, own account workers
5	Lower supervisory and technical
6	Semi-routine
7	Routine

Source: http://www.statistics.gov.uk/statbase/Product.asp?vlnk=8460

(c) Trends in life expectancy at birth in manual and non-manual occupational groups, England and Wales, 1972-2005

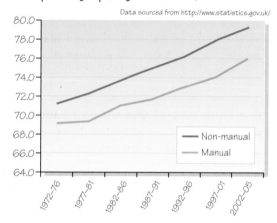

Data sourced from http://www.statistics.gov.uk/

— Non-manual
— Manual

(d) Differences in the probability of dying under the age of five between socioeconomic groups in three developing countries

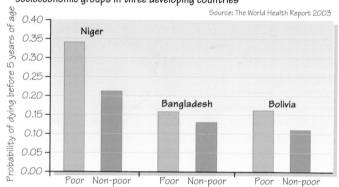

Source: The World Health Report 2003

Niger

Bangladesh

Bolivia

(e) Percentage of boys aged 2-15 years eating different types of food more than once a day by social class, England 1998

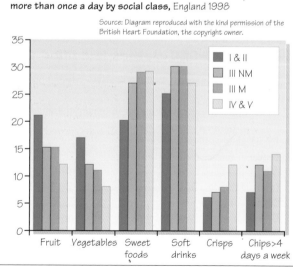

Source: Diagram reproduced with the kind permission of the British Heart Foundation, the copyright owner.

- I & II
- III NM
- III M
- IV & V

Fruit, Vegetables, Sweet foods, Soft drinks, Crisps, Chips>4 days a week

(f) Themes and principles in 'Tackling Health Inequalities: A Programme for Action'

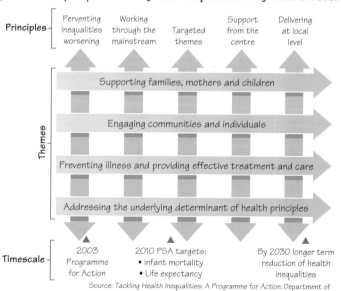

Principles — Preventing inequalities worsening · Working through the mainstream · Targeted themes · Support from the centre · Delivering at local level

Themes —
Supporting families, mothers and children
Engaging communities and individuals
Preventing illness and providing effective treatment and care
Addressing the underlying determinant of health principles

Timescale —
2003 Programme for Action
2010 PSA targets:
• infant mortality
• life expectancy
By 2030 longer term reduction of health inequalities

Source: Tackling Health Inequalities: A Programme for Action. Department of Health, London, 2003; PSA: public service agreement

Public Health and Epidemiology at a Glance, First Edition. Margaret Somerville, K. Kumaran, Rob Anderson.

In Chapter 19, we considered the variations in health status between population groups. Inequalities in health are nothing new. In the UK, Farr referred to the problem as early as 1860. Subsequently, the Black Report in 1980, the Acheson Report in 1998 and the Marmot Review in 2010 all highlighted persistent health inequalities and suggested priorities for action. While some factors affecting inequalities are unavoidable such as age, gender and genetic make-up, many other factors responsible for inequalities in health are related to social and economic inequalities in society and can be modified. There is evidence not only to confirm the presence of socio-economic inequalities in health but also to demonstrate that these inequalities are increasing. Figure 20a illustrates that the mortality rate in men belonging to social class V was 1.2 times greater than those in social class I in the early 1930s. This gap had increased to 2.9 times by the early 1990s. Figure 20b shows that there continues to be a clear gradient in the risk of death from the most advantaged group to the least advantaged group, with men in routine jobs having nearly three times greater age-standardised mortality rates than those in higher managerial posts.

Figure 20c shows trends in life expectancy at birth in manual and non-manual occupations between 1972 and 2005. While life expectancy has increased steadily in both groups (from 71.2 to 79.2 years in non-manual and 69.1 to 75.9 years in manual occupations), the gap between the two groups has increased from 2.1 years to 3.3 years. Currently life expectancy at birth between different electoral wards in the UK differs by over 10 years in both men and women.

These differences do not apply only to life expectancy or death rates. In the UK, the average difference in disability-free life expectancy between those living in the richest neighbourhoods compared to those living in the poorest neighbourhoods is 17 years. Therefore, not only do poorer people die sooner, they also spend more time living with a disability. Again, there is a gradient across the range with these patterns being seen in terms of education, housing, and other measures of social and economic status. Some of these factors are interrelated – for example, lack of education is associated with poor employment opportunities and consequently lower incomes. These socio-economic inequalities in health are not only observed in developed countries but can also be seen in developing countries (Figure 20d).

Health inequalities are linked to the conditions in which people are born and in which they live, consequently impacting on differences in opportunities, access to services, and lifestyle choices. These factors also have an effect on subsequent generations. Figure 20e shows that children born to parents in higher socio-economic groups tend to eat more fruit and vegetables and fewer sweets, soft drinks and crisps than children born to parents in lower socio-economic groups.

Inequalities in access to health care can be an important contributory factor to health inequalities. According to the **inverse care law** (Julian Tudor Hart 1971),

The availability of good medical care tends to vary inversely with the need for the population served. This inverse care law operates more completely where medical care is most exposed to market forces, and less so where such exposure is reduced. The market distribution of medical care is a primitive and historically outdated social form, and any return to it would further exaggerate the maldistribution of medical resources.

Tackling inequalities in health

From a public health perspective, the fact that avoidable inequalities exist between population groups is unfair and unacceptable in a developed society. However, tackling health inequalities is complex and requires coordinated action across agencies with multiple actions directed at both the health issues and the underlying socio-economic determinants of health to reduce the gap between different population groups and geographical areas.

In England, the importance given to tackling inequalities was demonstrated in 2003 by the Department of Health's strategy, 'Tackling Health Inequalities: A Programme for Action'. The strategy identified four themes and five principles for action which would reduce inequalities in the longer term (Figure 20f). The strategy also marked the setting of a national public service agreement (PSA) target to reduce inequalities in health outcomes by 10% as measured by infant mortality and life expectancy at birth by 2010.

More recently, the Marmot Review (2010) identified the most effective evidence-based strategies for reducing health inequalities from 2010 onwards. The review suggested that actions focusing on the most disadvantaged would not be sufficient but that to reduce the steepness of the socio-economic gradient in health inequalities, actions must be universal but with a scale and intensity that is proportionate to the level of disadvantage ('proportional universalism'). The report also highlighted the economic benefits of reducing health inequalities from increased productivity and tax revenue and decreased welfare payments and treatment costs. The report identified six main policy objectives that would help in reducing inequalities:
• Give every child the best start in life
• Enable all children, young people and adults to maximise their capabilities and have control over their lives
• Create fair work and good employment for all
• Ensure healthy standard of living for all
• Create and develop healthy and sustainable places and communities
• Strengthen the role and impact of ill-health prevention.

Delivering these objectives will require action at various levels by multiple organisations. The ultimate measure of success will be a fairer distribution of health and wellbeing across areas and different socio-economic groups.

21 Health needs assessment

(a) Model of health needs assessment

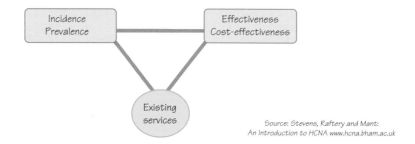

Source: Stevens, Raftery and Mant:
An Introduction to HCNA www.hcna.bham.ac.uk

(b) Outline of a possible HNA for alcohol-related harm

Components of an epidemiologically-based needs assessment	Example structure for a health needs assessment for alcohol-related harm
Size and nature of the problem	Patterns and amount of alcohol consumption Description and definition of alcohol use and misuse Prevalence of alcohol use disorders, injuries, maternal and perinatal conditions Alcohol-attributable mortality Alcohol-specific admissions to hospital and contacts with emergency services Specific high risk groups such as young people and the homeless Social impacts such as family breakdown, unsafe sex, effects on children Contribution of alcohol to crime and disorder such as violence and drink-driving Contribution of alcohol to inequalities in health
Effective and cost-effective interventions for prevention and treatment	Strategies for controlling the availability of alcohol such as taxation, price, licensing laws, minimum age drinking laws Strategies for reducing demand: educational programmes, unit labelling Strategies for problem limitation such as brief interventions to identify and counsel hazardous and harmful drinkers, stepped approach to treating alcohol misuse, programmes tailored to individual need, safety measures in licensed premises, breath-testing of drivers
Current services for prevention and treatment	Contribution of alcohol-specific conditions to general health service use such as emergency, primary, community and hospital-based care Specialist services for detoxification, dependency and treatment of acute and chronic alcohol-specific problems Other agencies' service provision such as diversionary schemes in the criminal justice system Voluntary agencies' provision e.g. support for problem drinkers and their families
Stakeholder engagement	General public, patients and their families and carers, voluntary agencies such as Alcoholics Anonymous, alcohol industry, police and criminal justice system, social work, health professionals
Recommendations	Most useful if specific recommendations are phrased as actions for individual services or agencies
Outcomes for monitoring progress	Alcohol-related and alcohol-specific mortality and hospital admissions Alcohol-related transport accidents Alcohol-related crime Outputs and activity from prevention and treatment services

Public Health and Epidemiology at a Glance, First Edition. Margaret Somerville, K. Kumaran, Rob Anderson.

Why should we assess health needs?

Health services have usually developed in response to a perceived need for them by either service users (i.e. the public) or providers (i.e. health professionals). Over time, populations and public expectations change, some diseases disappear, new diseases appear and medical knowledge and technology develops, so that prevention and treatment options also change. Services may or may not adapt to these changing patterns. As a result, using existing health service provision as an indicator of what is needed in terms of health care for a population can be very misleading. Health needs assessment provides a systematic way of assembling information to plan, negotiate and change health services for the better. Reducing inequalities in health should also be an explicit aim of health needs assessment and service provision.

Definition of need

Health needs assessments (HNA) are conducted to inform the development of services, so a health problem is only considered a health need if it can be addressed by an effective intervention or service provision. Such a need is described as 'normative' as it is defined by professionals rather than patients or the general public. An identified health need may be met by prevention or treatment services, by agencies other than health, or by wider social or environmental change. Health problems may generate demand for health services, influenced by patients' expectations of possible benefits or by health professionals' influence on patients, but demand does not necessarily indicate need.

need = ability to benefit from health care

HNA may be more precisely called **health care needs assessment (HCNA)**, but the terms are used interchangeably.

Epidemiologically based HNA

Various models for conducting HCNA have been developed, of which Stevens, Raftery and Mant's model (Figure 21a) has been widely adopted. The three main components of HCNA in this model are
- Size of the problem (incidence and prevalence)
- Review of the evidence for the effectiveness and cost-effectiveness of interventions and services
- Current service provision

Assembling data on incidence and prevalence is the **epidemiological and comparative approach** to HCNA, providing information on the size and nature of the condition under consideration (e.g. Figure 21b). For some common conditions or population groups, such as diabetes or older people, it may be appropriate to conduct a needs assessment at a local, small-scale level (locality or primary care centre), but for less common problems, or ones that require expensive, complex interventions, needs assessments are more appropriately undertaken at regional or national level.

Alongside the epidemiological information, evidence of what interventions are effective in the diagnosis, prevention and treatment of the condition or disease is essential for subsequent service planning and provision. High quality evidence reviews and evidence-based guidelines are now routinely available through organisations such as the Cochrane Collaboration and National Institute for Health and Clinical Excellence (NICE) in the UK, so minimising the need to undertake extensive literature searches at a local level. Evidence about the cost and cost-effectiveness of alternative interventions, however, may be more scarce and less conclusive.

Current service provision should also be described. Such a description should include the current workforce and levels of activity, such as numbers of clinics, consultations, admissions, operations and other procedures undertaken. Ideally the prevailing model of care delivery should be related to interventions or models of care in the evidence of effectiveness and cost-effectiveness. Views on the service should be sought from managers, staff and patients and also from other services, such as primary care, voluntary organisations or diagnostic facilities, that may refer patients in to the service or otherwise work with it. If big changes to services are anticipated, then formal consultation with such stakeholders, including with the public, may be needed. This **corporate** aspect of HNA may not always tally with the epidemiological or comparative data. Service users may have very different expectations of the service provided compared to the formal evidence base, while professionals may not be aware of some of the limitations of the current service, such as access for specific user groups, or only be concerned about certain specific aspects, such as specialist care for a minority of service users.

Finally, the HNA should provide a set of recommendations, ranked according to importance for implementation, for how the service should be provided, preferably after taking all views into consideration. The rate and extent to which recommendations can be implemented will depend on the resources available. Expectations about the level of resource that might be available, or other ways in which recommendations can be implemented, should be made clear before any work is undertaken. These different aspects and stages of HNA closely reflect the more generic stages of the 'planning cycle' (see Chapter 36). Finally, service changes should be evaluated and the HNA revisited to ensure that health needs continue to be met.

Rapid appraisal

Conducting a comprehensive HNA can be a major undertaking, particularly where specific surveys or other data collections are needed to fill gaps in routine data provision. If time or resources are not sufficient for a full HNA, then a rapid appraisal can give sufficient information on which to base planning decisions. A rapid appraisal uses qualitative research methods to capture knowledge and views of local health problems from communities and their leaders; it is a form of corporate HNA.

22 Disease prevention

(a) Concepts of disease causation and possible approaches to prevention: the natural history of disease

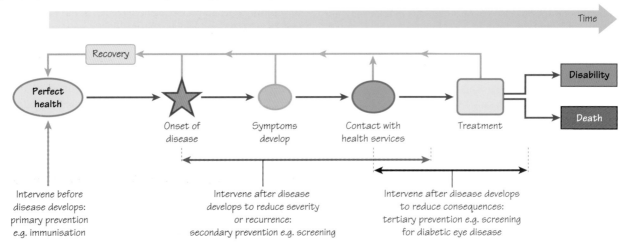

Time

Recovery

Perfect health → Onset of disease → Symptoms develop → Contact with health services → Treatment → Disability / Death

Intervene before disease develops: primary prevention e.g. immunisation

Intervene after disease develops to reduce severity or recurrence: secondary prevention e.g. screening

Intervene after disease develops to reduce consequences: tertiary prevention e.g. screening for diabetic eye disease

(b) The prevention paradox: the blue curve shows the frequency distribution of the risk factor, while the yellow line shows the risk of disease

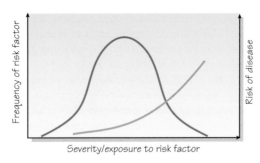

Frequency of risk factor / Risk of disease

Severity/exposure to risk factor

Increasing exposure to a risk factor, such as increasingly high levels of blood pressure, increases the risk of getting the disease caused by the risk factor, such as stroke

Only a small proportion of the population have very high levels of blood pressure, so only a small proportion are at very high risk of a stroke; many more strokes will occur in people with lower blood pressure levels

(c) High-risk versus universal approaches to prevention

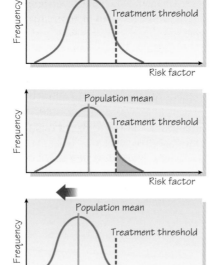

Population mean / Treatment threshold / Frequency / Risk factor

Risk factors such as blood presure levels and alcohol consumption are normally distributed through the population

Population mean / Treatment threshold / Frequency / Risk factor

Targeting prevention and treatment at those with the highest levels of risk will reduce individual risk but not contribute to substantial reductions in population risk

Population mean / Treatment threshold / Frequency / Risk factor

Adopting universal prevention measures shifts the population mean to the left, preventing more disease and reducing the proportion of people above the treatment threshold

Public Health and Epidemiology at a Glance, First Edition. Margaret Somerville, K. Kumaran, Rob Anderson.

Prevention is considered a good thing to aspire to: preventing a disease occurring in the first place is clearly preferable to treating it once it has developed. By adopting this approach, surely we must be preventing suffering and death and prolonging life? For an individual who is certain to develop a serious disease in the future, taking effective preventive measures now definitely seems worthwhile. In some cases, however, a disease may get better spontaneously without any treatment, may take a long time to develop or never cause serious problems during the lifetime of the affected individual. Taking preventive measures in these circumstances will not benefit the individual concerned and may cause harm, inconvenience or expense if those measures have side effects or involve lifestyle changes, taking long-term medication or regular tests such as radiographs.

Providing there is full information available on the potential benefits and risks of the preventive measures proposed, individuals can decide for themselves whether to follow them or take the risk of developing the disease. The balance of risks and benefits, however, is different for prevention compared with treatment for symptomatic disease; the benefit occurs in the future, while risks associated with the preventive measure occur now (e.g. taking antihypertensive medication to prevent strokes). At a population level, it may be necessary to apply preventive measures to many people, some of whom would never develop the disease in question, in order to prevent a few people dying or getting serious disease (e.g. compulsory wearing of car seat belts). This **prevention paradox** (Rose 2008) states that 'a preventive measure that brings large benefits to the community offers little to each participating individual'. Introducing disease prevention measures therefore needs careful consideration of the risks and benefits for individuals and populations.

The natural history of disease

In Figure 22a, the natural history of disease is shown as a simplified linear progression from perfect health. As the disease progresses, symptoms develop and, after a variable period of time, result in contact with health services and health professionals, leading to treatment. The outcome of treatment may be continuing disease and disability or death. At any point along this trajectory the disease may resolve, with an individual returning to health. Furthermore, at any stage, progression may be delayed by intervention.

- **Primary prevention** aims to prevent a disease developing in the first place. Immunisation (see Chapter 26) protects an individual from developing a specific communicable disease should they come into contact with it.
- **Secondary prevention** aims to reduce the severity or recurrence of a disease once it has developed. Screening (see Chapters 27 and 28) usually aims to identify and treat a disease in its early stages, before symptoms develop, thus reducing its severity and leading to a more complete recovery.

- **Tertiary prevention** aims to reduce the consequences of an established disease. Rehabilitation programmes following stroke reduce disability; screening for diabetic eye disease reduces the risk of blindness in those with established diabetes.

In practice, the boundaries between these categories are often blurred. The same preventive measures may be primary, secondary or tertiary depending on the populations they are applied to. For example, stopping children from smoking can be considered a primary prevention measure, as they are unlikely to have developed smoking-related disease. Stopping adults aged over 50, without any symptoms of smoking-related disease, from smoking can also be considered primary prevention, although it is likely that they would have some evidence of smoking-related disease if they were to be investigated. Stopping adults who have had a heart attack from smoking is secondary prevention, as they already have established ischaemic heart disease.

High risk versus population approaches

For most risk factors, the risk of disease increases with increasing exposure to the risk factor: for example, the higher an individual's blood pressure, the greater their risk of having a stroke (yellow line in Figure 22b). However, most risk factors such as high blood pressure or alcohol consumption are distributed through the population approximately normally (blue curve in Figure 22b). The people at highest risk of disease form a small proportion of those who actually develop it and most people who develop the disease do not have high levels of exposure to the risk factor. For example, most people who have strokes do not have very high blood pressure levels.

At an individual level, tackling those with the highest risk factor levels (e.g. those with the highest blood pressure levels) makes sense, as they are at the highest risk of developing disease (e.g. stroke). However, this targeted approach will not have much impact on the disease in the population as a whole, as the proportion of people at high risk is relatively small. It may be more effective to target the whole population to reduce levels of the risk factor. This population approach (Rose 2008) will have the effect of shifting the population mean of the risk factor to the left, reducing risk of disease in both the high risk group and the general population. Quite different preventive measures may be required for these two approaches: e.g. identifying and treating those with hypertension, or reducing salt consumption in the population as a whole through food industry regulation.

These two strategies are shown diagrammatically in Figure 22c. While more disease may be prevented by lowering risk in the whole population, rather than by reducing risk substantially in the small proportion at high risk, it may still be the case that only a minority benefit at an individual level.

Another model for disease prevention, the host–agent–environment model, is most frequently applied to communicable diseases and is discussed in Chapter 23.

23 Principles of disease transmission

(a) The epidemiological triad

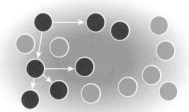

Factors affecting the epidemiological triad	
Host	Genetic susceptibility, immunity, nutrition, dose of pathogen received
Agent	Virulence, infectiousness, infective dose
Environment	Contact, overcrowding, vectors, reservoirs of infection, route of infection

(b) Illustration of reproductive number (R) in a totally susceptible population and in a population with 50% immunity
(Ro = basic reproductive number; R = net reproductive number; red circles = infected/diseased; apricot circles = susceptible; yellow circles=immune)

$R_0 = 2$ (on average) $R = 1$ (on average)

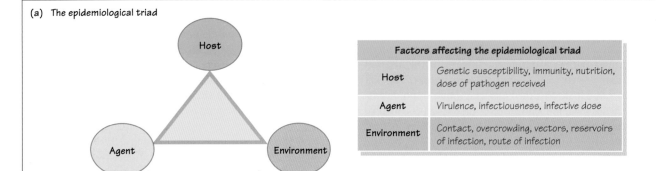

(c) Occurrence and patterns of disease (GP consultations for flu-like illness)

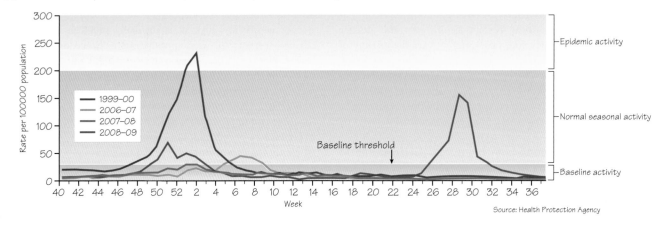

Legend:
- 1999–00
- 2006–07
- 2007–08
- 2008–09

Y-axis: Rate per 100000 population
X-axis: Week (40 42 44 46 48 50 52 2 4 6 8 10 12 14 16 18 20 22 24 26 28 30 32 34 36)

Baseline threshold

Epidemic activity
Normal seasonal activity
Baseline activity

Source: Health Protection Agency

(d) The chain of infection

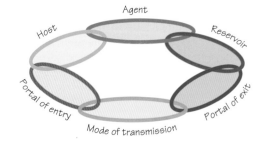

Host, Agent, Reservoir, Portal of entry, Mode of transmission, Portal of exit

Public Health and Epidemiology at a Glance, First Edition. Margaret Somerville, K. Kumaran, Rob Anderson.

The main determinants that influence disease transmission can be classified as the host, the environment, and the agent – commonly referred to as the **epidemiological triad**. The agent is the organism that causes the infection, the host is the potentially susceptible individual and the environment refers to the external factors that affect potential disease transmission. Figure 23a shows some of the key factors impacting on each of the three determinants.

Reproductive number

The transmission of a particular infection depends on a number of factors as outlined earlier. Key factors include the infection itself and the underlying population immunity. This is governed by the **reproductive number** (see Figure 23b). The **basic reproductive number** is the number of new cases that occur in a totally susceptible population. The **effective** or **net reproductive number** is the number of new cases that occur in a population where there may be both susceptible and immune people present. Mathematically, the net reproductive number is the product of the basic reproductive number and the proportion of susceptible individuals. For any infection to stop transmission, the effective reproductive number has to fall below 1: i.e. each case infects less than one person. This forms the principle of **herd immunity** (see Chapter 26). Although infections will tend to die out if the reproductive number is less than 1 on average, this assumes homogenous mixing patterns, where all instances of contact in the population are equally likely and therefore there is an equal chance for anyone to be potentially infected. In reality, mixing patterns are far from homogenous and transmission can therefore occur in groups where the reproductive number is greater than 1, even though the population average may be less than 1.

For example, even if herd immunity levels are reached for measles, it can continue to transmit in a group where the uptake of the measles, mumps and rubella vaccine (MMR) is low, e.g. travellers.

Routes of transmission

There are two main routes of transmission.
• Direct transmission:
  ◦ skin contact or touching, e.g. scabies
  ◦ sexual intercourse, e.g. syphilis
  ◦ droplet spread on to mucous membranes of the eye, nose or mouth by coughing or sneezing, e.g. influenza
  ◦ faecal–oral spread, e.g. gastrointestinal infections where faeces are transferred by direct contact
  ◦ transplacental, e.g. HIV
• Indirect transmission:
  ◦ contaminated fomites (clothing, bedding or other items in close contact with infected individuals), e.g. norovirus, influenza
  ◦ food or water, e.g. hepatitis A, cholera
  ◦ vectors, e.g. malaria
  ◦ blood borne, e.g. hepatitis B

Latent, incubation and infectious periods

The **latent period** is the time between infection and becoming infectious. The **incubation period** is the time between infection and becoming symptomatic. Obviously, if the latent period is shorter than the incubation period, it is more difficult to control the infection as it could potentially have spread before the index case shows symptoms and is diagnosed (e.g. influenza). The **infectious period** is the time during which an infectious agent may be transferred from

an infected person to another person. The length of these periods varies according to the infecting organism and the infective dose.

Consequences of exposure to infection

Once a person is exposed to an infection, the consequences, depending on the agent, may include:
• The infectious agent is eliminated without the host developing symptoms or becoming infectious.
• The infectious agent colonises the host (i.e. remains within or on the host without causing disease).
• The host develops an asymptomatic infection and can be infectious.
• The host develops a symptomatic infection and can be infectious.

Occurrence of infectious diseases

The occurrence of infectious diseases in a population are generally referred to as:
• **Sporadic:** occasional cases occurring irregularly
• **Endemic:** persistent background level of occurrence (low to moderate levels)
• **Epidemic:** occurrence in excess of the expected level during a given time period
• **Pandemic:** epidemic occurring in or spreading over several countries.

However, it is important to note that these terms may be applicable to the same disease in the same geographical area at different time periods. Similar levels of a disease that appears to be at epidemic level at one point may be considered 'normal' at another time period. For example, similar levels of seasonal influenza activity may be normal during winter, but considered an epidemic if occurring during summer (Figure 23c).

Principles of control

The spread of infection (or microorganism) from a source to a susceptible host is referred to as the **chain of infection** (Figure 23d). Control measures may therefore be aimed at various points along the chain of infection. If any of the links in the chain can be broken, the transmission of infection can be halted. Some key actions include:

Host factors

Direct protection of host by:
• Immunisation
• Prophylactic treatment
• Improved nutrition and general health.

Environmental factors

Prevent/reduce contact between agent and host:
• Barriers (personal protective equipment, condoms, bed nets)
• Reduce numbers of agent reaching potential host (hand washing, reduced overcrowding, food hygiene measures, sewage disposal, water treatment, control of vector numbers).

Agent factors

Reduce amount of agent released:
• Treat cases to reduce infectious period
• Isolate cases
• Eliminate/reduce environmental reservoirs.

(a) Management of single cases

Aims of managing single cases
- Identify the cause, source and mode of transmission of infection
- Look for links to potential sources or to other cases
- Stop further transmission or spread
- Ensure case is appropriately managed
- Protect contacts at risk

Key issues to consider in managing cases
- Risk assessment
- Modes of transmission
- Control measures

(b) Epidemic curves for an organism with an incubation period of 2-10 days (median 5–6 days).

(i) **Point source epidemic**

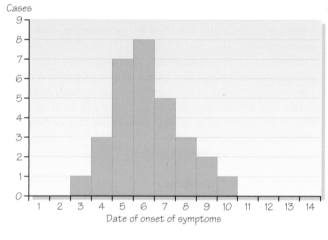

(ii) **Continuous source epidemic**

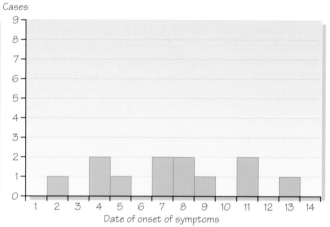

(iii) **Person-to-person spread epidemic**

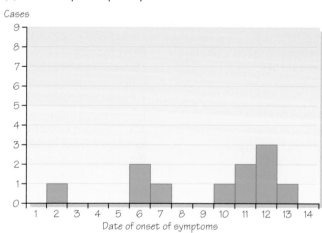

Public Health and Epidemiology at a Glance, First Edition. Margaret Somerville, K. Kumaran, Rob Anderson.

Managing single cases of communicable diseases (Figure 24a)

The following issues need to be considered in assessing risk:
• Who is at risk?
• From what?
• How is it spread?
• What control measures are necessary?
• Who/what are the sources of advice?
• Where are the policies and guidelines?

Individual control measures that can be used include:
• Removal of the source of infection if possible
• Treatment of the case as appropriate to reduce infectivity
• Isolation/exclusion as necessary
• Prophylaxis to close contacts (drugs, vaccine, immunoglobulin).

Case studies
Antibiotic prophylaxis to close contacts to prevent transmission

Meningococcal disease is spread from person to person requiring close contact for transmission to occur. Close contacts of an infected individual are therefore offered antibiotic prophylaxis to: prevent disease if they are not incubating it already, and eradicating meningococcal carriage to prevent further transmission.

Immunisation to contacts to prevent transmission

Hepatitis B is usually transmitted via infected body fluids or transplacentally. In the case of an infected pregnant woman, her newborn child is offered a course of immunisation after birth (with or without immunogloblin) to prevent disease.

Isolation and treatment of the case to prevent transmission

Influenza can be infectious even before the onset of symptoms making control of infection difficult. Isolation measures and antiviral treatment of the case reduces infectivity and the length of the infectious period.

Exclusion of the case to prevent transmission

Causes of gastrointestinal disease, resulting in diarrhoea and/or vomiting and abdominal pain, are many and varied. Some tend to be self-limiting, while others are potentially more dangerous. Excluding those who are at high risk of transmitting infection such as food handlers and health and social care staff will reduce transmission. The general recommended period of exclusion is 48 hours after the cessation of symptoms.

Universal precautions

It is not always possible to identify people who may be infectious, so there are certain precautions that should be followed at all times, especially in health and social care settings. These are generally referred to as universal precautions, and include:
• Good basic hygiene with regular hand-washing – the single most important aspect of infection control
• Covering wounds or skin lesions with waterproof dressings
• Use of appropriate personal protective equipment to deal with the risk of potentially infected body fluids
• Safe disposal of sharps and knowing what to do if there is an inoculation injury
• Cleaning of contaminated surfaces and safe disposal of contaminated waste

• Cleaning, disinfection and sterilisation of equipment as appropriate.

Outbreaks
Definition

An outbreak can be defined as:
• Two or more people who experience a similar illness or confirmed infection, and are linked by a common factor, or
• When the observed number of cases unaccountably exceeds the expected number for a given place and time.

The term can be used to describe a range of situations from local outbreaks of food poisoning to international epidemics. The terms epidemic and outbreak are used interchangeably.

Management

Procedures include:
• Confirmation of the outbreak (i.e. ensuring it is real and not an artefact)
• Identification of the causative organism, its source and mode of transmission
• Removal of the source if possible
• Interruption or prevention of transmission
• Ensuring cases receive treatment
• Ensuring that lessons learnt lead to appropriate modifications to policy and practice.

Factors that influence management include:
• Nature of disease, e.g. single case of polio in a polio-free area
• Number of cases, e.g. diarrhoea and vomiting affecting a large school
• Setting in which infection arises, e.g. residential care home, local community
• Commonly used and widely available product implicated, e.g. cryptosporidium in public water supply.

In the UK, outbreaks with significant public health implications are managed by a formal outbreak control team.

First, the problem should be confirmed and the diagnosis verified. Control measures may have to be instigated immediately to stop further transmission based on the initial available information, as preventing further cases of disease takes precedence over investigating the cause or source.

The initial epidemiological approach involves active case finding, as the initial cases discovered may only be the most severely affected. A clear case definition is required. Data are then collected usually using standard questionnaires to generate an initial hypothesis. This descriptive epidemiology allows us to describe cases by time, place and person. Plotting an epidemic curve, a frequency distribution of date of onset, may identify an incubation period which, combined with clinical features, can help identify the potential cause and source of spread: e.g. point source, continuous source, person-to-person spread (Figure 24b).

The initial hypothesis can then be tested or confirmed by conducting analytical epidemiological studies, usually a case-control or cohort study (see Appendix), which may involve further microbiological or environmental tests. Further control measures may then be necessary. Surveillance is necessary to determine when the outbreak control team can declare the outbreak over, using agreed preset criteria. Finally, any lessons identified should be used to help prevent future outbreaks.

25 Surveillance

(a) (i) The purpose of surveillance

- Individual case management to prevent spread
- Recognition and control of outbreaks
- Detect emergence of new infections
- Measure change in incidence
- Track change in risk factors
- Evaluation of control measures
- Influence health policy

(ii) The principles of surveillance

- Case definition
- Case identified using a variety of data sources
- Dataset collected for each disease and case
- Analysis of data
- Interpretation of information
- Dissemination and **action**
- Continuing surveillance

(b) The Iceberg Effect: only a small proportion of cases are confirmed

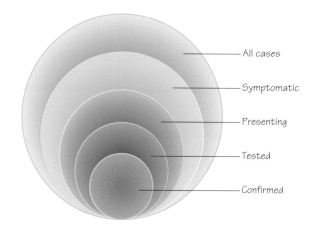

- All cases
- Symptomatic
- Presenting
- Tested
- Confirmed

(c) (i) Late detection and response

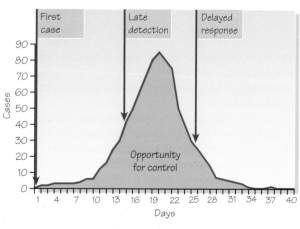

(ii) Early detection and response

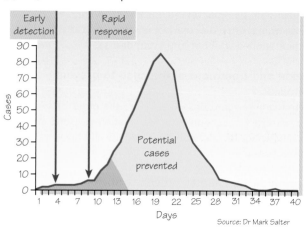

Source: Dr Mark Salter

(d) Laboratory reports of invasive haemophilus influenzae type b (Hib), England and Wales, 1990-2005

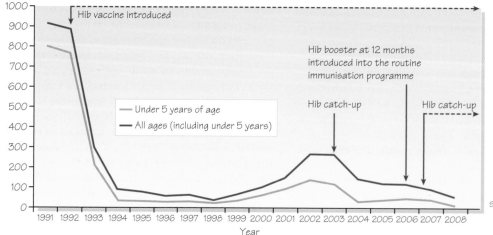

Source: Health Protection Agency

Public Health and Epidemiology at a Glance, First Edition. Margaret Somerville, K. Kumaran, Rob Anderson.

Definition

Surveillance has been defined as the continuing scrutiny of all aspects of the occurrence and spread of a disease that are pertinent to effective control. It involves a systematic collection, collation and analysis of data and the prompt dissemination of the resulting information to those who need to know so that **action** can result (Figure 25a).

Although this chapter focuses on surveillance of communicable diseases, the principles apply similarly to non-communicable diseases including cancers.

Sources of data for surveillance

In the UK, there is a statutory requirement for certain infectious diseases to be notified by registered medical practitioners to public authorities. This originally dates from the late 19th century, but the legislation has been revised recently to provide public authorities with new powers and duties to prevent and control risks to human health. In addition to the list of infectious diseases, the new regulations require clinicians to notify public health authorities of cases of other infections or contamination (including chemical or radiation) that could potentially be a significant risk to human health.

Other sources of surveillance data in the UK include the weekly returns from the Royal College of General Practitioners, NHS Direct (a 24-hour nurse-led telephone service in England and Wales), QSurveillance (a collaborative national project which captures primary care data), enhanced surveillance systems for specific infections of public health importance, Medical Officers of Schools Association and the British Paediatric Surveillance Unit (of the Royal College of Paediatrics and Child Health). Data on sexually transmitted infections is usually obtained from genitourinary medicine clinics. International surveillance data is obtained from the World Health Organization.

Principles of surveillance

The basic principles of surveillance are listed in Figure 25a. An ideal surveillance system needs to be:
- Continuing
- Practical
- Consistent
- Timely
- Accurate
- Complete.

It is important to keep in mind that the number of confirmed cases is usually only a small proportion of the total cases in the community (Figure 25b). The proportion of true cases that are identified will vary depending on the severity of the infection – for example, most cases of meningococcal meningitis will present to health services, but many cases of diarrhoea due to norovirus will not.

Example: Surveillance to detect a new infection

Using the H1N1 swine flu pandemic of 2009 as an example, consider the development of a surveillance system for an emerging/new infection.

After WHO issued a global alert about the spread of swine flu in Mexico and the USA, it was important for cases to be promptly recognised in the UK so that appropriate control measures could be instigated. Figure 25c demonstrates the difference that early recognition and action can make in preventing cases.

First, we need a case definition to identify cases of swine flu in the UK. It is much easier to detect an infection that is already known than to try and detect a new infection. The case definition in the initial stages necessarily has to be sensitive, so that all possible cases are recognised and measures can be put to place to try and control the spread of the infection. The case definition will usually consist of a combination of clinical features and epidemiological features. The epidemiological component will relate to symptoms occurring within the incubation period after returning from an affected area. It can also relate to onset of symptoms within the incubation period in a close contact of a known case.

While the early recognition of cases can help to prevent spread, it is important during the early stages that the diagnosis is confirmed using specific microbiological tests. The surveillance system needs to be designed to enable necessary actions, which include:
- Early treatment of cases (to reduce severity and to stop transmission)
- Interruption of transmission to close contacts such as health care workers and household members by appropriate measures
- Collection of information to enable better understanding of the virus and its spread.

The surveillance system needs to consider collecting data from a number of sources including clinicians, laboratories and additional sources such as schools, pharmacies and ports of entry. It is essential that the case definition is widely disseminated and reporting mechanisms are quick, easy and practical to ensure good response rates.

Once the infection becomes well established, it may be appropriate to stop or change special surveillance systems based on clinical or public health need. However effective action based on the development of an active surveillance system initially helps to delay the potential spread and allows time for the development of a vaccine.

Example: surveillance to monitor the effectiveness of public health interventions

Figure 25d illustrates the fall in *Haemophilus influenzae* type B (Hib) notifications following the introduction of the Hib vaccine, with a rise from about 1999 onwards. Analysis by time, place and person showed that the rise was observed across England and Wales between 1999 and 2003. While children under the age of 5 were mostly affected in the pre-vaccine era, the recent rise was observed both in the under-5s and in older age groups. Vaccine coverage rates remained high. Serological surveys suggested that immunity tended to wane if the vaccine was given only during infancy; however if the vaccine was given after the first year of life, immunity tended to last longer. This finding led to a change in the immunisation programme with an additional dose being offered after 1 year of age. Subsequently, the number of cases began to decline again after the introduction of the booster dose.

(a) Characteristics of live and killed vaccines

Live vaccine:	
Advantages	**Disadvantages**
Strong immune response	Potential to revert to virulence and may cause disease occasionally
Single dose often results in life long immunity	Poor stability
Frequency of adverse reactions decreases with number of doses	Most live vaccines contraindicated in immunosupressed individuals

Killed vaccine:	
Advantages	**Disadvantages**
Good stability	Need several doses
Unable to cause disease	Shorter immunity
Can be given to immunosupressed individuals	Local reactions more common and frequency of adverse reactions increase with number of doses

(b) The principle of herd immunity

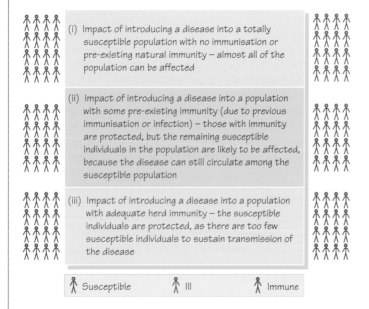

(i) Impact of introducing a disease into a totally susceptible population with no immunisation or pre-existing natural immunity – almost all of the population can be affected

(ii) Impact of introducing a disease into a population with some pre-existing immunity (due to previous immunisation or infection) – those with immunity are protected, but the remaining susceptible individuals in the population are likely to be affected, because the disease can still circulate among the susceptible population

(iii) Impact of introducing a disease into a population with adequate herd immunity – the susceptible individuals are protected, as there are too few susceptible individuals to sustain transmission of the disease

Susceptible   Ill   Immune

(c) The current UK National Childhood Vaccination Programme (January 2011)

Age	Vaccine
2 months	DTaP/IPV/Hib & PCV
3 months	DTaP/IPV/Hib & Men C
4 months	DTaP/IPV/Hib & Men C & PCV
12–13 months	Hib/Men C & MMR & PCV
Pre-school	DTaP/IPV or dTaP/IPV & MMR
School leaver	Td/IPV

Note:
HPV is given only to girls aged between 12–13 years
BCG is given only to those considered at high risk
D = Regular dose diphtheria
d = Low dose diphtheria
aP = acellular Pertussis
T = Tetanus
IPV = Polio
PCV = Pneumococcal
Hib = Haemophilus influenzae b
Men C = Meningococcus Group C
MMR = Measles, mumps, rubella
HPV = Human papilloma virus
Note: See www.who.int for immunisation schedules of all countries

(d) Whooping cough cases in England and Wales and vaccine coverage in England, 1940–2005

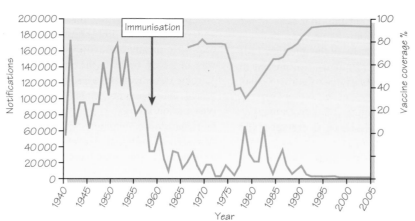

Vaccination coverage, England only
Source: Health Protection Agency

Immunisation is an example of primary prevention and is one of the most effective public health interventions. Immunisation refers to the process of developing immunity to certain diseases by injecting antigens or serum containing specific antibodies. Although the terms vaccination and immunisation are now used interchangeably, vaccination in the strict sense of the term refers to the process of inoculation using cowpox (vaccinia) to prevent smallpox.

Although the mechanisms are complex, there are essentially two broad categories of immunity: innate or non-specific immunity, and acquired immunity.

Innate or non-specific immunity refers to the natural immunity possessed by individuals without prior exposure to a specific antigen.

Acquired immunity can be either active or passive:
• **Active immunity** involves the production of specific antibodies either after natural exposure to disease or after artificial inoculation by vaccines. Specific antibodies are produced against an antigen resulting in persistent immunological memory.
• **Passive immunity** is provided by the administration or transfer of antibodies; it provides temporary protection and is usually used when individuals are at high risk of developing disease.

Vaccines can be developed using either live or killed organisms. Figure 26a lists the advantages and disadvantages for each type of vaccine.

Some individuals fail to produce an adequate immune response to an initial course of the vaccine (primary vaccine failures). For example, about 10% of the population fail to produce an adequate response to the measles component of the MMR vaccine. Occasionally, an individual produces an adequate response initially but then immunity wanes over a period of time (secondary vaccine failure). This can happen particularly with killed vaccines; further doses are required to boost immunity.

Herd immunity

Herd immunity is the concept that an individual who is susceptible to an infection may still be protected against that infection if sufficient numbers of people in the community are immune to it. The concept only applies to infections transmitted solely by person-to-person spread. The proportion of the population needing to be immune in order to confer protection on the remaining susceptible individuals is referred to as the **herd immunity threshold**. This depends on the effective reproduction number (see Chapter 23) for the relevant infection and is achieved when each case of the infection is transmitted to less than one other person. When this stage is reached, the infection cannot be sustained in the community and is eliminated (Figure 26b).

Example: measles transmission

If each case of measles can infect 15 susceptible individuals, then to prevent increasing spread of the disease, at least 14 of every 15 people in the population need to be immune either by immunisation or through natural immunity. Therefore the percentage of the population that needs to be immune is 14/15 = 93%. Taking into account that about 10% of the population may not develop adequate immunity to a single dose of vaccine, we will need to immunise about 95% of the population with two doses of vaccine to ensure adequate herd immunity levels.

Development of an immunisation programme

The aims of any immunisation programme are to contain, eliminate or eradicate risk (universal immunisation e.g. national childhood immunisation schedule), or to protect those at highest risk (selective immunisation, e.g. BCG and hepatitis B) from disease. Effective surveillance can help to estimate the disease burden and to decide on the appropriate strategy. Once a vaccine is introduced, surveillance should be continued to monitor vaccine effectiveness as well as adverse reactions. In the UK, recommendations on introducing an immunisation programme are made by the Joint Committee on Vaccinations and Immunisations (JCVI). The UK national childhood immunisation schedule is shown in Figure 26c.

Internationally, the campaign to eradicate smallpox has been the most successful immunisation programme: WHO declared smallpox to have been eradicated worldwide in 1979 after the last case occurred in Somalia in 1977. It remains the only vaccine-preventable disease to have been eradicated globally. Global eradication of polio may be close; although large parts of the world are now polio free, it continues to be of concern in parts of Asia and Africa.

Perceptions of risks and benefits of immunisation programmes

After an immunisation programme is well established and herd immunity levels have been achieved, with a consequent decline in rates of disease, the benefit of immunisation to a given individual decreases. When perceived risks from immunisation are highlighted, rates of vaccine coverage can decline especially if people perceive the disease as not significant. Figure 26d shows a decline in vaccine coverage in the UK during the early 1970s as a result of a fear of neurological sequelae from the pertussis (whooping cough) vaccine. The coverage improved again after the initial reports were proven to be unfounded but not before an increase in the number of cases occurred, with some deaths from whooping cough, during that period.

There are obvious public health and ethical implications related to mass immunisation programmes. If overall immunisation rates are adequate, then an individual refusing immunisation may still be protected because of the herd immunity effect. However, immunisation is recommended for all, as individual refusals do ultimately have an impact upon whether herd immunity is achieved and maintained. When herd immunity is not achieved, it can have major health impacts, and particularly so for those who cannot be immunised for medical reasons (and who may have otherwise been protected due to herd immunity). The perception that vaccine-preventable diseases are mild is incorrect, as all cause serious illness (seen less and less frequently in countries with effective immunisation programmes), although some may cause milder illnesses in some individuals. Therefore, immunisation remains important at both an individual and population level.

(a) **The natural history of disease:** as assumed by screening principles, showing disease progressing from its onset, through stages at which it is asymptomatic but can be identified by testing, to symptomatic disease, the normal clinical diagnostic and treatment process and either recovery, continued disease or death. The lower part of the diagram shows the altered course of the disease if screening occurs, picking up the disease at an earlier stage, resulting in earlier treatment and improved outcome.

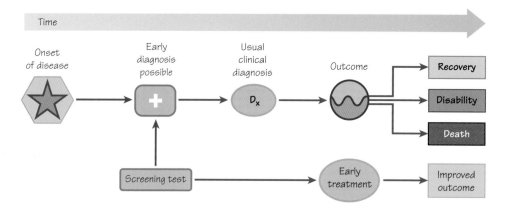

(b) **Lead time bias:** the two upper arrows indicate the length of survival from diagnosis either with or without screening. The difference between the two is the lead time bias.

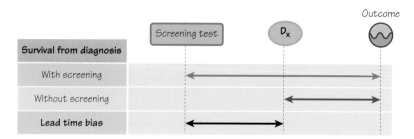

(c) **Length time bias:** for slowly progressive disease, there is plenty of time for the screening process to pick up the cancers, but there is less time for rapidly progressive disease to be picked up. The latter cancers may therefore be missed by the screening process.

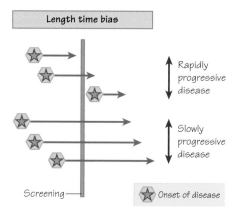

Public Health and Epidemiology at a Glance, First Edition. Margaret Somerville, K. Kumaran, Rob Anderson.

60 © 2012 John Wiley & Sons, Ltd. Published 2012 by John Wiley & Sons, Ltd.

Screening is usually considered a form of secondary disease prevention, as it aims to reduce morbidity and mortality from a disease, rather than preventing the disease altogether. The benefits of screening arise from early diagnostic testing and treatment compared with usual symptomatic ('late') diagnosis and treatment (Figure 27a). Some screening tests and programmes, however, pick up precursors of a disease, rather than the disease itself; treating the disease precursors may prevent the disease occurring in the first place. An example is screening for cervical cancer, where the screening test picks up precancerous changes which can then be treated, thus preventing progression to cancer. Other screening tests and programmes pick up conditions that cannot be prevented, particularly genetically determined ones such as Huntington's disease, when the aim of screening is to provide information for those affected.

Definition of screening

The UK National Screening Committee currently defines screening as:

> A process of identifying apparently healthy people who may be at increased risk of a disease or condition. They can then be offered information, further tests and appropriate treatment to reduce their risk and/or any complications arising from the disease or condition.

Assumptions

Screening is generally thought to be a 'good thing' as it is appealing to think that, if a disease is picked up at an early stage, treatment is more likely to prevent serious illness developing and may lead to cure (Figure 27a). However, it is important to realise that this intuitive understanding of screening is based on several assumptions:
• That the natural history of the disease is well known, that it has a latent phase when it can be identified before the person is aware of any symptoms for which they would normally seek health advice, and that progression from that latent phase to serious disease is highly probable.
• That there is an appropriate test available to accurately identify those with latent disease and to exclude those without the disease.
• That effective treatment for early disease is available and that treatment at an early stage leads to better outcomes for the person compared to treatment following presentation with clinical symptoms.
• That no one will be harmed by the test, the treatment or the screening process.

Certain criteria must therefore be met before implementing any screening programme to ensure that it is more likely to produce more benefit than harm (see Chapter 28).

Screening tests

Screening tests should ideally be very sensitive, so that very few people with the disease are missed (false negatives) and also very specific, so that very few people without the disease are identified for further investigation and treatment (false positives). In reality, no screening test is perfect and there is a trade-off between sensitivity and specificity to be made. It is also important to remember that, when screening is carried out on an unselected general population, disease prevalence is usually low. Most people who test positive in these circumstances will therefore not have the disease being tested for (see Chapter 11).

Example

In the pilot programmes for bowel cancer screening in England, only 10% of those undergoing further investigation following a positive faecal occult blood test were found to have bowel cancer.

Ethical considerations

Screening is unlike standard health care, where an individual seeks contact with health services because of symptoms or concerns about their health. In contrast, screening programmes, by definition, are offered to people who do not think they have the disease in question and have not therefore sought health advice. For those people who accept an offer of screening, some who do not have the disease may test positive (false positives) and then undergo further testing and treatment unnecessarily, to their detriment. Others may have asymptomatic disease and are not identified by the screening test (false negatives) and are then falsely reassured that they have no cause for concern. For these reasons, people who are offered screening must be fully informed of the possible benefits and harms.

Sources of bias in assessing screening programmes

Lead time bias is the time by which diagnosis is advanced because of screening (Figure 27b), which leads to an apparent increase in survival.

Example

A person is going to die from bowel cancer at the age of 62. He or she develops symptoms and is diagnosed at the age of 61, so their survival from diagnosis is 1 year. If he or she had been picked up with asymptomatic disease on screening at the age of 59, their survival would be 3 years, but as death still occurs at the same age, there is no difference in the outcome.

Length time bias: diseases with a long latent phase are more likely to be picked up by screening than those with a short latent phase (Figure 27c).

Example

Some prostate cancers are very slow-growing and may take many years before causing symptoms, if they ever do, while others develop quickly and cause serious disease over a short time span. There is therefore a smaller window of opportunity for any screening test for prostate cancer to identify the rapidly progressive cancers in time to treat them effectively.

Volunteer bias: those who accept invitations to be screened tend to be those at lower risk of the disease ('healthy screenees') and healthier generally. If a screening programme has poor coverage of its target population, then it is likely that those who would benefit most from screening are being missed.

Example

In the New York Health Insurance Plan trial, an RCT of screening for breast cancer in 300 000 women over 5 years, the death rates from causes other than breast cancer were similar between those offered screening and those not offered screening. Those who accepted the invitation and were screened, however, had half the death rate of those who did not accept (42.5 vs 85.6 deaths per 10 000 women) (Shapiro 1977).

(a) General flow diagram for any screening programme

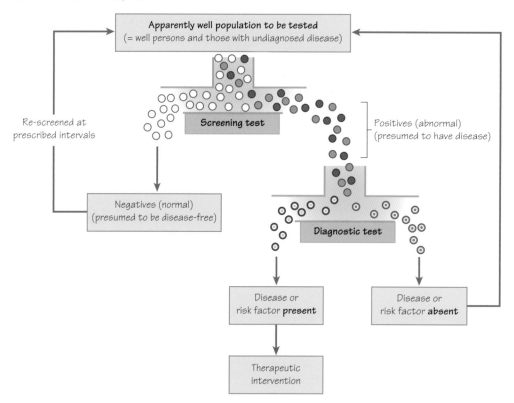

Apparently well population to be tested
(= well persons and those with undiagnosed disease)

Screening test

Re-screened at
prescribed intervals

Positives (abnormal)
(presumed to have disease)

Negatives (normal)
(presumed to be disease-free)

Diagnostic test

Disease or
risk factor **present**

Disease or
risk factor **absent**

Therapeutic
intervention

(b) Flow diagram for the UK breast screening programme. The cancer detection rate in 2008-9 was 7.8 per 1000 women screened

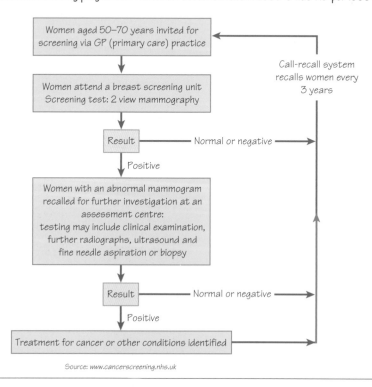

Women aged 50–70 years invited for
screening via GP (primary care) practice

Women attend a breast screening unit
Screening test: 2 view mammography

Result — Normal or negative →

Call-recall system
recalls women every
3 years

Positive

Women with an abnormal mammogram
recalled for further investigation at an
assessment centre:
testing may include clinical examination,
further radiographs, ultrasound and
fine needle aspiration or biopsy

Result — Normal or negative →

Positive

Treatment for cancer or other conditions identified

Source: www.cancerscreening.nhs.uk

Public Health and Epidemiology at a Glance, First Edition. Margaret Somerville, K. Kumaran, Rob Anderson.

Screening may be undertaken proactively, by systematically inviting everyone in a specified target population for screening over a defined time period. The UK breast screening programme, for example, invites all women aged 50–69 years for a screening test (mammography) once every 3 years.

Screening may also be undertaken opportunistically, when a person seeks help for another problem. Those attending emergency departments following an injury, for example, may be screened using a questionnaire to determine if they are drinking alcohol at a hazardous level.

Elements of a screening programme

A population-based screening programme consists of more than a screening test (see Figure 28a for a generic flow diagram of any screening programme and Figure 28b for a simplified flow diagram for the UK breast screening programme). Follow-up investigations for those who test positive must be defined and available within a reasonable time. Effective treatment must be available for those who remain positive after further investigation. Staff must be trained to perform screening tests and further investigations, provide appropriate evidence-based advice on risks and benefits, and deliver treatment for those with the condition. The information conveyed to participants in a genetic screening programme requires particularly careful communication and provision of supporting advice (e.g. genetic counselling). Genetic test results may also have disease risk or reproductive planning implications for other family members, not just the person screened.

There must be explicit quality standards for delivery of the programme and an administrative system for inviting people to be screened, communicating results and referring on appropriately.

Criteria for appraising the viability, effectiveness and appropriateness of a screening programme

To avoid introducing ineffective screening programmes, the Wilson and Jungner criteria, originally set out in a WHO report in 1948, are used to assess the extent to which new screening programmes could be expected to be effective in reducing harm from the disease in question. The UK National Screening Committee now applies these criteria to proposals for new programmes. Ideally, all should be met before a new screening programme is introduced.

The condition
• Should be an important health problem.
• The epidemiology and natural history of the condition, including development from latent to declared disease, should be adequately understood and there should be a detectable risk factor, disease marker, latent period or early symptomatic stage.
• All cost-effective primary prevention interventions should have been implemented as far as practicable.
• If the carriers of a mutation are identified as a result of screening the natural history of people with this status should be understood, including the psychological implications.

The test
• Should be simple, safe, precise and validated.
• Should be acceptable to the population.
• The distribution of test values in the target population should be known and a suitable cut-off level defined and agreed.

• There should be an agreed policy on the further diagnostic investigation of individuals with a positive test result and on the choices available to those individuals.
• If the test is for mutations, the criteria used to select the subset of mutations to be covered by screening, if all possible mutations are not being tested, should be clearly set out.

The treatment
• There should be an effective treatment or intervention for patients identified through early detection, with evidence of early treatment leading to better outcomes than late treatment.
• There should be agreed evidence-based policies covering which individuals should be offered treatment and the appropriate treatment to be offered.
• Clinical management of the condition and patient outcomes should be optimised in all health care providers prior to participation in a screening programme.

The screening programme
• There should be evidence from high-quality randomised controlled trials that the screening programme is effective in reducing mortality or morbidity. Where screening is aimed solely at providing information to allow the person being screened to make an 'informed choice' (e.g. Down's syndrome, cystic fibrosis carrier screening), there must be evidence from high-quality trials that the test accurately measures risk. The information that is provided about the test and its outcome must be of value and readily understood by the individual being screened.
• There should be evidence that the complete screening programme (test, diagnostic procedures, treatment/ intervention) is clinically, socially and ethically acceptable to health professionals and the public.
• The benefit from the screening programme should outweigh the physical and psychological harm (caused by the test, diagnostic procedures and treatment).
• The opportunity cost of the screening programme (including testing, diagnosis and treatment, administration, training and quality assurance) should be economically balanced in relation to expenditure on medical care as a whole (i.e. value for money). Assessment against these criteria should consider evidence from cost benefit and/or cost effectiveness analyses and the effective use of available resource.
• All other options for managing the condition should have been considered (e.g. improving treatment, providing other services), to ensure that no more cost-effective intervention could be introduced or current interventions increased within the resources available.
• There should be a plan for managing and monitoring the screening programme and an agreed set of quality assurance standards.
• Adequate staffing and facilities for testing, diagnosis, treatment and programme management should be available prior to the commencement of the screening programme.
• Evidence-based information, explaining the consequences of testing, investigation and treatment, should be made available to potential participants to assist them in making an informed choice.
• Public pressure for widening the eligibility criteria, reducing the screening interval, and increasing the sensitivity of the testing process, should be anticipated. Decisions about these parameters should be scientifically justifiable to the public.
• If screening is for a mutation, the programme should be acceptable to people identified as carriers and to other family members.

29 Health promotion

(a) Areas of health promotion action as set out in the Ottawa Charter for Health Promotion (www.who.int)

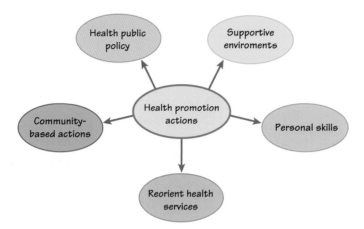

(b) Examples of tobacco control actions and the levels and settings at which they work, based on NICE public health guidance (www.nice.nhs.uk) and UK Tobacco Control policies (www.dh.gov.uk)

Levels of intervention	Example: tobacco control
Personal skills	Stop smoking interventions: brief advice to stop smoking, nicotine replacement therapy, self-help materials
Community actions	Media campaigns on tobacco-related harm linked to other activities such as policy changes or school-based interventions Warnings on cigarette packets
Supportive environments	No smoking policies on public transport, in public buildings Campaigns promoting smoke-free homes and cars Restricted and regulated tobacco sales points Legislation preventing tobacco sales to children
Healthy public policy	High tax on tobacco products Smoking bans in public places Advertising and sponsorship bans
Reorient health services	Preventive and intensive support services e.g. group behaviour therapy, individual behavioural counselling, telephone counselling and quitlines Stop smoking services targeted at high-risk groups, e.g. pregnant women

Public Health and Epidemiology at a Glance, First Edition. Margaret Somerville, K. Kumaran, Rob Anderson.

What is health promotion?

In 1986, the Ottawa Charter defined health promotion as:

the process of enabling people to increase control over, and to improve, their health. To reach a state of complete physical, mental and social well-being, an individual or group must be able to identify and to realise aspirations, to satisfy needs, and to change or cope with the environment. Health is, therefore, seen as a resource for everyday life, not the objective of living. Health is a positive concept emphasising social and personal resources, as well as physical capacities. Therefore, health promotion is not just the responsibility of the health sector, but goes beyond healthy life-styles to well-being.

Range of health promotion activities

Promoting health can be undertaken in many ways and in many settings. Health promotion can focus on intervention at the individual level; through health education initiatives and provision of support to encourage behaviour change; this support necessarily also involves changes at a wider environmental level. Whole populations may be the focus of promotional interventions such as local or national campaigns and programmes, as well as legislative interventions including taxation. Health promotion is delivered through the actions of a range of organisations; local and national government, health services, schools and businesses, and through community groups. These actions can be organised at a number of geographical levels, from neighbourhood to national level.

The Ottawa Charter identified five areas of health promotion activity (Figure 29a); Figure 29b shows how these areas can be applied to tobacco control. Other models of health promotion have been developed, including the community development approach, which has led to the Healthy Cities movement, developed by the WHO, which:

seeks to promote comprehensive and systematic policy and planning for health and emphasises:

• the need to address inequality in health and urban poverty
• the needs of vulnerable groups
• participatory governance
• the social, economic and environmental determinants of health.

This is not about the health sector only. It includes health considerations in economic, regeneration and urban development efforts (www.who.int)

Health promotion programmes

A health promotion programme should be based on assessment of need and evidence of the effectiveness of what is proposed. Otherwise, where there is an important health need but a lack of evidence, a decision needs to be made about whether there is a good theoretical rationale for expecting the programme to influence practice. A programme should have a stated aim with specific objectives, involve implementation of one or more well-defined, evidence-based interventions, delivered to a specified target population in a particular setting, with clearly defined outcomes. Specifying outcomes needs to include both immediate and longer-term outcomes; the ultimate aim of a tobacco control programme may be to reduce tobacco-related illness and death, but it takes a long time for changes in these diseases to become apparent. This lengthy timeframe makes it difficult to attribute any changes to a specific time-limited intervention. Shorter-term outcomes can, however, also be defined, including self-reported measures of behaviour change, although less reliable than objectively measured outcomes. On the other hand, process measures, such as the numbers of posters displayed or programme participants in a given time period, may be valuable to indicate that a programme was carried out as intended, but gives no indication of whether any health or behaviour change occurred as a result of the activity.

Example: a programme to promote smoke-free homes and cars

Rationale:	Following the bans on smoking in public places in the UK, exposure to second-hand smoke (SHS) in the non-smoking population fell, but children of parents who smoked still experienced major exposure to SHS in private homes and cars which are not subject to the ban. Children exposed to SHS are more likely than children not exposed to SHS to suffer from respiratory illness
Aim:	To reduce the exposure of children with parents who smoke to SHS
Objectives:	To raise awareness of the risks of SHS To persuade adult smokers to commit to keeping their homes and cars partly or wholly smoke-free
Target population:	Children with parents who smoke; adults who smoke and have children
Settings:	Schools; media; fire and rescue services
Interventions:	School-based activities, including educational sessions and competitions National and local media campaigns Information and campaigns run by fire and rescue services Community networks promoting smoke-free as the norm
Process measures:	Numbers of parents and other adults signing up to keep their homes and cars smoke free Numbers of signs displayed on cars declaring their smoke-free status
Outcomes:	Numbers of children exposed to SHS in the home or car Prevalence of respiratory illness in children of parents who smoke Smoking-related house fires

Source: *Healthy Lives, Healthy People: A Tobacco Control Plan for England*. Department of Health, 2011.

Models of behaviour change in (a) individuals (b) and (c) communities (d) organisational working (adapted from Nutbeam D. *Theory in a Nutshell*)

(a) Transtheoretical model of behaviour change in individuals

Precontemplation

Contemplation
Acknowledging that there is a problem but not yet ready or sure of wanting to make the change

Relapse
Returning to older behaviours and abandoning the new changes

Preparation
Getting ready for change

Maintenance
Maintaining the behaviour change

Action
Changing behaviour

Stable behaviour

(b) Behaviour change in communities: diffusion of innovation

Percentage of adopters / Time

Laggards 10–20%
Late majority 30–35%
Early majority 30–35%
Early adopters 10–15%
Innovators 2–3%

(c) Behaviour change in communities: dimensions of community organisation and capacity-building

Addressing problems / Building strengths / External/expert driven / Community driven

Local government moves community to new housing estate because existing housing is inadequate

Local residents lobby for improvements to existing housing, which is cold and damp

National scheme awards funding to a community for redevelopment

A rural community sets up and runs a local shop

(d) Ways organisations work together

Full collaboration
Coalition
Partnership
Alliance
Network

Written agreement, joint budget, shared decision-making, formal work programme

Loose association, no formal commitments

Public Health and Epidemiology at a Glance, First Edition. Margaret Somerville, K. Kumaran, Rob Anderson.

Improving the health of populations ultimately means that individuals, communities and organisations need to change their behaviour to become healthier. Health promotion programmes are more likely to be successful if their interventions are based on theories of behaviour change, of which there are many. Some of the most commonly used theories are briefly summarised below.

Health education

Health professionals are usually very keen to provide patients and the public with information and advice on healthy behaviour. Such enthusiasm leads to the production of leaflets, posters, campaigns and other methods of raising people's awareness and knowledge of health risks and healthy lifestyles, from what constitutes a healthy diet to warnings about catching AIDS. Providing such information in accessible formats is essential, but is not enough on its own to reliably produce behaviour change, which is strongly influenced by external, environmental and social factors.

Working with individuals

The **knowledge–attitudes–behaviour (KAB)** model is one approach to changing behaviour in individuals; knowledge of a health risk and how to avoid or minimise it is expected to change behaviour towards a more healthy lifestyle. There is a well-recognised gap, however, between knowledge of a health risk and taking action to avoid it, well illustrated by smoking: few people openly deny that smoking is harmful to health, but a substantial proportion of the population continues to smoke on a regular basis. The **health belief** model suggests that people will change their behaviour to avoid a specific risk to their health if they believe that the risk is serious, that they themselves are likely to get the condition and that there is action they could take to avoid or minimise the risk, the benefits of which outweigh the costs.

The **transtheoretical model** (Figure 30a) has been used extensively to encourage behaviour change. In the UK, the stop smoking services have been very successful in using this model, first to identify smokers who would like to stop smoking and then to support them in preparing to stop, setting a date to stop (a quit date) and providing practical help, such as nicotine replacement treatment, to maintain their non-smoking status. Similar steps can be used to help people with behaviour change in other situations, such as reducing alcohol consumption.

Working with communities

Communities are more than collections of individuals; they have their own capabilities and dynamics that require consideration if healthy change is to be achieved. The **diffusion of innovation** theory (Figure 30b) describes how a new idea is adopted in a community. Innovators, a small proportion, take it up most quickly, followed by the early adopters. They are followed by the early and late majorities, the bulk of the community, and finally, the laggards, some of whom may never adopt the innovation. Health-promoting innovations are more likely to be adopted if they clearly offer an advantage over existing practice, are compatible with the community's social and cultural values, are fairly simple, flexible and reversible and the beneficial results of adopting the innovation are made evident to those who may be thinking of adopting it.

Community development can also be seen along a spectrum of participation and empowerment, from interventions decided by 'experts' external to the community which are then carried out without consultation to those generated by the community itself with no outside support. Interventions may also be focused on specific immediate problems, such as traffic, noise or pollution, or may be aimed more at building sustainable long-term capacity for the community to tackle what it perceives as its own priorities (Figure 30c).

Working with organisations

Organisations can be seen as communities in some respects; the diffusion of innovation theory can be very useful when introducing new ideas or ways of working into complex organisations such as health services. Equally important, however, is the way in which organisations work together. Health promotion often requires action to be taken across agencies; for example, health services and local government may need to work with private business and voluntary organisations to ensure that the local population has easy access to leisure and exercise facilities or cheap convenient transport. Organisations can work together in a variety of ways (Figure 30d), with increasingly formalised collaborative decision-making and work programmes.

Working with policy-makers

The development of healthy public policy is a key aspect of health promotion. Those involved in policy-making include the politicians and bureaucrats or civil servants who formulate the policies, the lobby groups and others who seek to influence the policy-makers, the media and the public, who will finally determine the extent to which a policy is actually adopted.

Social marketing

Social marketing is a recently developed health promotion activity which recognises the techniques of commercial marketing firms and their ability to target audiences for specific products with the intention of increasing sales. These marketing techniques are now being applied to selling health, by identifying key target groups, understanding their culture and motivation and then using the information to tailor health promotion interventions to appeal to that particular audience.

The scope of health economics

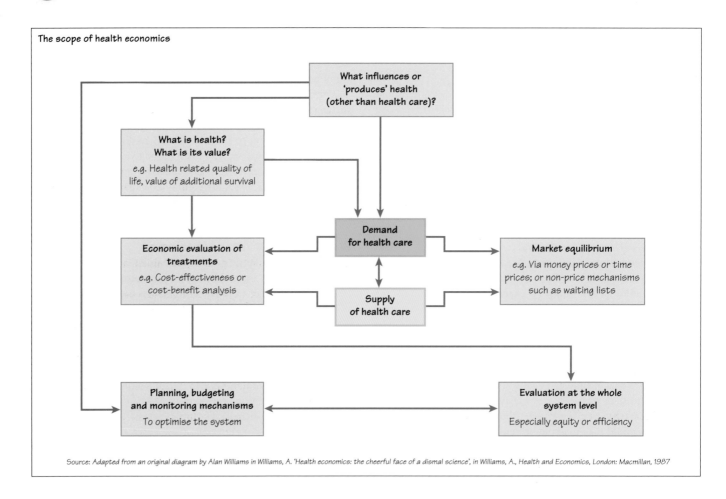

Source: Adapted from an original diagram by Alan Williams in Williams, A. 'Health economics: the cheerful face of a dismal science', in Williams, A., Health and Economics, London: Macmillan, 1987

Public Health and Epidemiology at a Glance, First Edition. Margaret Somerville, K. Kumaran, Rob Anderson.

68 © 2012 John Wiley & Sons, Ltd. Published 2012 by John Wiley & Sons, Ltd.

Dr David Kernick, a general medical practitioner from Exeter, in England, has said:

> Life in healthcare organisations is a continuum of decisions on how physical and human resources are allocated. Against a background of limited budgets, resources invested into one area are at the expense of a lost opportunity in another and difficult decisions are inevitable. Every decision in healthcare is a rationing decision. Expanding one service means that there is less for another, an extra five minutes spent with one patient will be at the expense of the next.

This is a useful introduction to health economics for two reasons. First, it clearly describes one of the most useful concepts of economics and health economics – **opportunity cost**. For economists, the true cost of a good, a service or a treatment is not the specific amount of money that was paid for it. Instead, the true cost of something is the value of the benefits foregone by not applying the same money or resources to the next best alternative. This is because most decision-making, in health care or elsewhere, takes place under conditions of scarcity. Scarcity of resources, in turn, necessitates choices – you can't have everything. And choices nearly always imply opportunity costs.

Secondly, it reminds us that all decisions in healthcare – and doctors make or influence a great many of them – are resource-allocating decisions. While much of medicine is said to be about making 'clinical decisions' (i.e. decisions made about patients by or with health professionals), all such decisions usually also commit resources and therefore have opportunity costs.

What is economics?

If health economics is the application of the theory and methods of economics to health and health care, what is economics? Although studying 'the economy' – for example, the performance of national economies – forms a part of the subject of economics (macro-economics), the discipline of economics covers a great deal more. Many non-economists find economics a daunting subject because it is often so highly mathematical, and so highly theoretical, that it seems more like a branch of physics or philosophy.

Economics can be variously described as the 'science of choice', the 'science of incentives', or the study of 'how markets work'. Among the social sciences, economics has been criticised for being over-reliant on explanations based on self-interest and rational behaviour; that is, that individuals make choices only based on what will improve their own wealth and satisfaction. At the same time its core concepts of opportunity costs and the analysis of costs versus benefits involved in choices, and an understanding of how supply and demand interact for different goods or services, provide important ways of understanding many areas of human endeavour including health, health care and medicine.

A quick guided tour of health economics

Although Figure 31 tries to provide a comprehensive overview of the subject of health economics, the breadth of the subject can also be shown by the wide range of questions that health economists might ask. For example:
• Will an increase in tax on cigarettes be of overall benefit to society?

• Does paying doctors on a fee-per-service basis mean that patients get more treatment than they need?
• How should changes in quality of life be measured and valued?
• Is it cost-effective to screen more frequently, or using a more accurate but more costly test?
• How do economic factors (such as income levels, unemployment, food prices, public transport provision) impact upon healthy eating, physical activity and obesity?
• Would investing money in reducing social inequalities improve the health of more people than a population-level health promotion programme?

These are just some of the many interesting questions which health economists ask, and which they have developed methods to try to answer. As well as the traditional economic focus on explaining demand and supply, and equilibrium in markets, the subject includes interest in philosophical and epidemiological questions such as how to value life, and how factors beyond health services such as income and education influence health.

Health economics and health systems

Much of the subject of economics is about how and whether markets 'work', that is whether they are the best way to meet society's goals. Markets are generally believed to work best – to be a so-called 'perfect market', matching and meeting society's goals with available resources – when there is perfect information about demand and the goods available, when suppliers can enter or leave the market easily, and various other conditions. Economists then explain how markets work by defining various departures from this idealised model of reality.

The market for healthcare is highly unusual because it fails at a number of levels. For example, unlike normal markets for many other goods, patients have to rely on someone else – the doctor, acting as their 'agent' – to help decide what they need. Also, in some situations people get satisfaction or value from other people receiving health care (for example, if the rest of a community receive vaccination).

Most importantly, though, a person's need for health care is highly unpredictable – we generally don't know when we will be ill or how seriously ill we may be in the future. For all these reasons, in most developed countries health care is mostly funded collectively, through taxation or national health insurance. Other markets related to health care, for example the supply of doctors and nurses, are often also quite highly regulated because free and 'perfectly competitive' markets generally do not exist in the field of health.

Health economics, resource allocation and efficiency

Given widespread recognition of 'market failure' in health care, and therefore considerable government intervention, the methods of health economics have had an increasingly important role in planning health care and public health policy. This is because economics provides useful methods for assessing the relative efficiency of organisations (such as hospitals) or proposes rational approaches to resource allocation and priority-setting in health systems. However, the methods of economic evaluation, to establish which treatments or health programmes provide the best value for money, or are the most cost-effective, are probably the most widely used by health economists (see Chapter 32).

Economic evaluation

(a) The basic elements of an economic evaluation

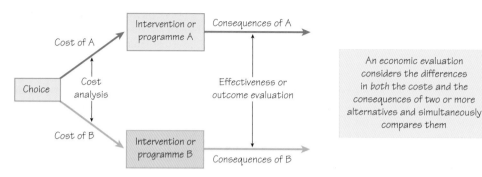

An economic evaluation considers the differences in both the costs and the consequences of two or more alternatives and simultaneously compares them

(b) The three main types of economic evaluation

Cost-benefit analysis	Outcomes expressed as health and other benefits are measured, valued in monetary terms, and costs are then deducted (e.g. £ or $)	Results expressed as Net benefit, in £s or $s (if positive, benefits exceed costs,a then intervention ashould be implemented)
Cost-effectiveness analysis	Outcomes are expressed in 'clinical units'	£ or $ per case detected, per life-year saved, or per acute episode avoided
Cost-utility analysis	Outcomes are expressed in terms of quality-adjusted life-years (QALYS) or Disability-Adjusted-Life-Years (DALYs)	£ or $ per QALY gained

(c) Possible policy implications of cost-effectiveness results of a new compared with an existing treatment or programme
An incremental analysis involves comparing the additional costs invested/saved with the additional effectiveness gained/lost. If the results fall in the grey-shaded areas of the table, other considerations – beyond cost or effectiveness – may become important, and also the magnitude and certainty of any expected cost savings or effectiveness gain.

		Effectiveness difference		
		Less effective	Same effectiveness	More effective
Cost difference	More costly	NO! Don't invest in the new treatment		Conduct an 'incremental analysis'*
	Same cost			
	Less costly	Conduct an 'incremental analysis'*		Yes! invest in the new treatment

Public Health and Epidemiology at a Glance, First Edition. Margaret Somerville, K. Kumaran, Rob Anderson.

Doctors, health service managers and policy-makers clearly want to provide treatments and services which are safe, effective and acceptable to patients. It is less obvious but also critical that they are cost-effective – that is, that they represent good 'value for money' for the health system or society as a whole. In the language of the previous chapter, it is important that the benefits exceed the opportunity costs. Thus the rigorous assessment of the balance of benefits and costs – or economic evaluation, as it is more broadly known – is a major strand of the work of health economists.

A policy-maker's concern about the cost and cost-effectiveness of a treatment typically has another element though, affordability. While cost-effectiveness is to do with judging the desirability of a particular decision, affordability is about whether there are enough resources available; for example; can a hospital or the health system afford the total cost?

What is an economic evaluation?

Economic evaluation is simply the comparative evaluation of *both* the costs and the effects of *two or more alternatives* – such as alternative treatments, health services or public health programmes. As well as measuring the effectiveness of alternative treatments an economic evaluation would also require measurement of the costs of using the treatment (Figure 32a).

However, an economic evaluation does not just capture the costs of initially providing the treatments. If the treatment is effective, and improves health, then there may be reduced or delayed health care costs (e.g. due to fewer acute episodes, such as asthma attacks, or a reduced need for monitoring appointments or supporting medication). Therefore, a good economic evaluation will normally assess the costs and effects of a treatment for a number of years – preferably for as long as either the costs or the effects are likely to differ between the compared alternatives.

Three main types

In health care, three main types of economic evaluation are used: **cost-benefit analysis**, **cost-effectiveness analysis**, and **cost-utility analysis**. However, the term cost-effectiveness analysis is also sometimes used as a general term covering all these methods. Costs will generally be measured and valued in the same way for each of these approaches. They are distinguished from each other by the way they measure and value health impacts (see Figure 32b).

Which of these methods is appropriate for any given choice will depend on the exact nature of the targeted condition, the degree to which alternative treatments affect quality of life (as opposed to survival) and whether there are significant impacts of the treatment on broader social, education or other non-health outcomes. Although in principle cost-benefit is the most comprehensive and ideal form of economic evaluation, the practical difficulties and ethical concerns raised by valuing health in monetary terms mean that the other two approaches – cost-effectiveness and cost-utility analysis – have become more widely used in the health field.

Cost-benefit analysis

Cost-benefit analysis involves the valuation of all benefits and costs in monetary terms, and is believed by health economists to be the most theoretically well-grounded of the three main methods. It is also more likely to be used to evaluate public health interventions which have a broad range of both health and non-health impacts. For example, road injury prevention schemes may lead to health outcomes (such as more active travel and reductions in road casualties). But there might also be important impacts on the environment (noise and emission reductions), and important gains in the leisure and social value of having less congested streets around schools – which could all be valued and added in to the benefit–cost comparison. Housing regeneration may also have positive impacts beyond health, such as reducing crime and unemployment. These diverse outcomes could only be captured and combined by a cost-benefit analysis.

Cost-effectiveness analysis

Cost-effectiveness analysis has been used widely to assess whether the additional benefits gained by a new programme or treatment are worth the additional costs. Different screening policies for life-threatening diseases, such as cervical cancer, can be assessed in terms of the (additional) cost per (additional) life-year saved for progressively more costly and effective screening policies. For example, compared to no screening, the annual national cost of three-yearly cervical screening might be £1.5 million and thereby save an additional 100 women's lives per year. This would mean that the incremental cost per life-year saved of the three-yearly cervical screening programme is £15 000 per life-year saved. In other words, a cost-effectiveness analysis estimates the ratio of the additional (or incremental) costs to the additional benefits of a pair of alternatives.

Such 'incremental analyses' are important, since there is *always* an alternative policy or programme which would otherwise be implemented (even if it is occasional unplanned testing). Cost-effectiveness is an inherently relative concept, and nothing can 'be cost-effective' without reference to some alternative way of investing resources. Figure 32c shows the different policy implications that a cost-effectiveness analysis may create.

Cost-utility analysis

Cost-utility analysis is merely cost-effectiveness analysis in which the outcome estimated and compared between alternatives is the number of additional quality-adjusted life-years (QALYs). QALYs combine the two dimensions of survival and health-related quality of life (see full definition in Chapter 34). Since cost-benefit analysis in health is so difficult, and because so very few diseases or public health problems have an impact *only* on quality of life or *only* on survival, cost-utility analysis is the most commonly used method of economic evaluation in health care, and increasingly used to evaluate public health interventions. The main advantage of cost-utility analysis is that the number of QALYs gained by investing in alternative public health programmes, for different diseases, or invested in preventive versus curative care, can all be readily compared.

Using the results to inform policy

When comparing the costs and the effects of two alternative treatments, there is a range of possible results (see Figure 33c). Given that the cost of a new treatment may be higher, or lower, or the same as the current treatment, and that similarly the effectiveness of the new treatment may be assessed to be greater, worse or the same as the old treatment, there are nine alternative types of result that a policy-maker may have to interpret. For an alternative that is both more costly and more effective than another, policy-makers sometimes use an implicit cost-effectiveness threshold (e.g. £30 000 or $100 000 per QALY gained) above which most treatments or programmes would be deemed as 'not cost-effective'.

33 Economic perspectives on measuring health-related outcomes

(a) Survival and quality-adjusted survival

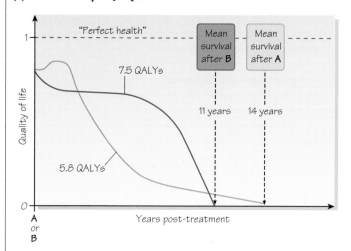

Table 33.1 Leading causes of the global burden of disease in 2004

	Disease or injury	DALYs (millions)	Percentage of total DALYs
1	Lower respiratory infections	94.5	6.2
2	Diarrhoeal diseases	72.8	4.8
3	Unipolar depressive disorders	65.5	4.3
4	Ischaemic heart disease	62.6	4.1
5	HIV/AIDS	58.5	3.8
6	Cerebrovascular disease	46.6	3.1
7	Prematurity and low birth weight	44.3	2.9
8	Birth asphyxia and birth trauma	41.7	2.7
9	Road traffic accidents	41.2	2.7
10	Neonatal infections and other	40.4	2.7

Source: The Global Burden of Disease, 2004 Update (WHO, 2008), Table on p.43

(b) Overview of three health state preference assessment techniques

1. Rating scales and visual analogue scales

Present respondents with a list of numbers (e.g. 0 to 10), or a line marked 0 at one end and 10 at the other (see below). 0 is labelled as 'health state as bad as being dead'; 10 is marked as 'full health'

0 (dead) ———————————— 10 (full health)

Respondents should choose a number, or mark the line, to represent precisely where between full health and 'zero health' they perceive the described health state to be.

2. Time Trade-Off (TTO)

Respondents are asked to choose between a certain number of years in the described disease state, and a lower number of years in perfect health (both followed by immediate death). The number of years in full health is varied until the respondent has equal preference for both options (i.e. when they would switch choice).

30 years in the described health state
or
x (i.e. fewer) years in full health

The preference weight for the described health state would then be calculated as $^x/30$

3. Standard Gamble

Respondents choose between spending the remainder of their lives, with certainty, in the described health state (option B, below), or another option (A) where there is a varying probability of either attaining full health for the remainder of their lives, or dying immediately. This time, finding the probability (P) under option A of gaining full health at which options A or B are equally preferred allows calculation of a preference weight for the option B health state.

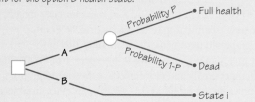

(c) Questions of the EQ-5D health-related quality of life questionnaire

By placing a tick in one box in each group below, please indicate which statements best describe your own health state today

Mobility
I have no problems in walking about	☐
I have some problems in walking about	☐
I am confined to bed	☐

Self-Care
I have no problems with self-care	☐
I have some problems washing or dressing myself	☐
I am unable to wash or dress myself	☐

Usual Activities (e.g. work, study, housework, family or leisure activities)
I have no problems with performing my usual activities	☐
I have some problems with performing my usual activities	☐
I am unable to perform my usual activities	☐

Pain/Discomfort
I have no pain or discomfort	☐
I have moderate pain or discomfort	☐
I have extreme pain or discomfort	☐

Anxiety/Depression
I am not anxious or depressed	☐
I am moderately anxious or depressed	☐
I am extremely anxious or depressed	☐

Source: EQ-5D. © EuroQol Group

Public Health and Epidemiology at a Glance, First Edition. Margaret Somerville, K. Kumaran, Rob Anderson.

Health economists have made significant contributions to the development of methods for measuring and valuing health outcomes. This chapter gives a brief overview of some of the most common measures now used (QALYs and DALYs) either in evaluating public health interventions or in prioritising investment for different global health problems, and also introduces the main methods used for valuing health states.

Quality-adjusted life-years (QALYs)

It is obvious that many diseases, and their treatments, affect **quality of life** (or morbidity) as well as **length of life** (or survival, mortality). In the last two decades various methods have emerged for combining both of these outcomes in the same measure. **Quality-adjusted life-years** (QALYs) count the number of years of 'full health' or 'perfect health' that would be equivalent to a greater number of years in a state worse than full health. For example, 10 years lived at 'half full health' would yield 5 QALYs, whereas 30 years at two-thirds full health would yield 20 QALYs.

The importance of the QALY is best illustrated by the graph shown in Figure 33a. After one treatment (A: let's say surgery) a patient lives on average for 14 years. This compares with only 11 years average survival following the medical treatment, B. On the basis of differences in survival, clearly treatment A would be preferred to treatment B. However, this ignores possible differences in the quality of life following treatment. In particular, while there is a slight rise in the quality of life following surgery, overall the quality of life following surgery is lower than that following medical treatment. In fact, for the last 3 or 4 years of added survival the quality of life is only marginally above zero (where zero is usually defined as 'as bad as being dead'). Patients obtain more QALYs after treatment B than treatment A.

Disability-adjusted life-years (DALYs)

Unlike QALYs, which were developed to support economic evaluations, **disability-adjusted life-years** (DALYs) were developed to assess the relative burden of different diseases and injuries (see also Chapter 16). Although both QALYs and DALYs are on the same scale (0 to 1), with DALYs 1 is death and 0 is full health/no disability, so a higher amount of DALYs represented a larger burden of disease. There are a number of other important differences, for example:
• The life-expectancy in DALY calculations is constant, and set at the national life-expectancy of Japanese women (i.e. the maximum attainable globally). QALYs can be calculated using any life-expectancy data.
• The 'disability weights' are based on person trade-off scores (see next section) from a sample of health care workers, rather than preference weights.
• The DALY has age-related weightings which give lower weights to young and elderly people.

DALYs were developed by the World Health Organization and have been used by WHO and the World Bank to assess which diseases, which causes of injury and which countries account for the most burden of disease (see Table 33.1).

Methods for valuing health states

Figure 33b describes three of the main techniques which are commonly used for eliciting preferences for different health states relative to full health: rating scale, time trade-off and standard gamble. For each method, a sample of respondents (e.g. 1000 randomly sampled members of the general public) are first presented with a description of a particular health state (including, the presence or absence of pain, impacts on physical wellbeing and social functioning, ability to perform normal daily functions. etc.). They are then presented with a choice, as described.

All three methods can produce a valuation of a health state between 0 and 1. The resultant values are often called 'utility weights' or simply utilities. Although more complicated, the standard gamble approach is generally preferred by health economists as it presents a choice with uncertainty, which is believed to be both more realistic and more compatible with the relevant economic theory.

Others have argued that the person trade-off method (as used for DALY weights) is superior because it aims to identify the number of people experiencing two different outcomes that would be regarded as equivalent value (suffering). It therefore has greater similarities with actual resource allocation decisions in populations.

Generic quality-of-life questionnaires

The health states which are valued can either be described in paragraphs of text (vignettes) or in quality of life questionnaires. The most widely used questionnaire for assessing health-related quality-of-life is probably the EQ-5D (or EuroQol) questionnaire, which asks people to assess their problems relating to mobility, self-care, usual activities, pain and/or discomfort, or anxiety and/or depression (see Figure 33c).

Given these five questions, each with three possible levels of response, there are 243 different health states that can be described by the EQ-5D. The preference weight for each of these health states has been estimated using a large survey of the general public in the United Kingdom (using the Time Trade-Off method). Some example social preference weights for different states are shown in Table 33.2. Note that many of the health states involving both severe problems and extreme pain/discomfort have been valued with negative scores. This means that they have been judged as being 'worse than death'.

There are also other health state classification systems that have produced social preference weights. The Health Utilities Index (HUI-2 and HUI-3) and the SF-6D (which is derived from SF-36 quality of life questionnaire responses) are the better-known ones. With more questions than the EQ-5D, they are able to capture other dimensions of health such as 'vitality' or sensory impairments, and in the case of the SF-36 provide separate scores for physical and mental health status. There is considerable debate about the reliability and validity of these different measures, and while the SF-36 and EQ-5D are now commonly used in clinical studies, their limitations should always be considered. Older quality of life questionnaires, such as the Nottingham Health Profile, were generally not designed either to generate a summary score or to have valuations calculated for different health states.

Table 33.2 EQ-5D social preference weights

Health state*	EQ-5D social preference weight
11111	1.000 (i.e. full health – no problems on all dimensions)
22111	0.746
12312	0.381
32133	-0.390

*1 represents having no problems, 3 represents extreme problems (or unable to be mobile, unable to perform self-care etc.), and 2 represents having some problems or moderate pain or anxiety, etc.

The complex causes of obesity related to food production

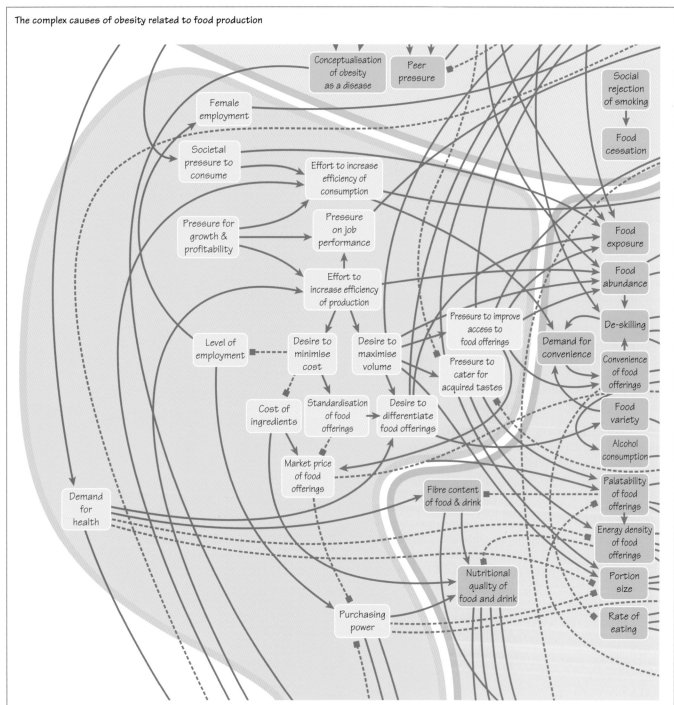

Source: Selected portion of the Obesity Systems Map from Foresight Tackling Obesities: Future Choices Project 2007. © Crown Copyright. www.foresight.gov.uk.

Notes: The right-hand column of factors shows some of the more direct aspects of the availability of different types of food, healthy or unhealthy, while the cluster of factors in the middle of the Food Production domain are driven by efforts to increase the efficiency of production. The combined impact of economic pressures to produce food more efficiently (cheaply) and social pressures to consume lie at the heart of the economics of food production and its role in creating obesity.

Public Health and Epidemiology at a Glance, First Edition. Margaret Somerville, K. Kumaran, Rob Anderson.

74 © 2012 John Wiley & Sons, Ltd. Published 2012 by John Wiley & Sons, Ltd.

The work of many health economists is to inform choices between alternative ways of treating health problems (i.e. economic evaluation, Chapter 32). Economic concepts and methods of analysis, however, may also help explain the underlying causes of various public health problems.

This chapter provides an overview of some of the arguments that economists have put forward to explain the substantial growth in obesity rates in recent decades. It then also examines the economic case for government intervention in reducing levels of obesity and overweight. There are also parallels in using economics to explain public health problems such as smoking or heroin addiction.

The economics of obesity

Almost all advanced industrialised countries are experiencing unprecedented growth in the prevalence of obesity – being overweight relative to a person's height. As well as having a direct impact on morbidity, obesity and being overweight increases the risk of developing a wide range of other diseases such as type 2 diabetes, heart disease and stroke.

While the fundamental cause of obesity is physiological, with individuals consuming more calories over time than are expended, the pattern of development of obesity in populations is determined by a range of genetic, environmental, social and behavioural factors. These might include increased car use, TV viewing, availability of fast food outlets, production of processed foods (typically high in salt and fat) and the proportion of women in the workforce (affecting the demand for convenience foods).

Health economists have contributed to understanding the causes of the 'obesity epidemic' largely through arguments relating to the impact of technological changes on how (and what) we eat, and whether (and how much) we exercise.

How technology may be fattening

Overall, in most countries, technological innovation in agricultural production has reduced the price of consuming calories. Technological innovation in other workplaces has also led to a much larger proportion of the workforce having sedentary, physically less active jobs (e.g. desk-based). This second change has two further impacts. First, fewer calories are expended during a normal day's work. Second, because exercise must then be taken during leisure time, the opportunity cost of expending calories increases.

There have also been technological changes in food preparation, such as packaging, use of preservatives, and microwave ovens, which have probably reduced the price of foods. Importantly, these price reductions include both the amount of money paid for food and also the **time costs** of preparing food in the home (i.e. opportunity cost of food preparation in terms of lost leisure time). From these assumptions it can be predicted, and some US evidence confirms, that the growth in consumption of calories in developed countries is associated not with more calories being consumed at meal times, but with more snacks between meals.

Economics can also help explain the social patterning of obesity within countries. Within most advanced economies, poorer people are more likely to be overweight or obese than those in higher income households. One economics-based reason for this might be that, in such countries, physical exercise has become an activity which usually has to be paid for, either in terms of sports club or gym subscriptions, or foregone leisure time. By having both a lower disposable income and often also fewer non-work hours, the less well off effectively pay a higher price for exercising.

In summary, economics, and in particular the key concept of opportunity cost, can provide plausible explanations for the rapid growth of obesity in developed countries. By examining the impact of technological changes on both **supply-side factors** (such as the production cost of food) and **demand-side factors** (such as the rise of time-poor households) economic explanations may also provide insights into potential policy solutions. For example, if the relatively low price of high-calorie pre-prepared meals is a key cause of the obesity problem (and given that governments pay most of the health care costs of obesity-related problems), then taxing fast foods may be a solution worth considering. Some of these economic factors affecting diet also emerged as important in a major recent exercise to understand the causes of obesity as a complex system (*The Foresight Report*: see Figure 35). Study the flow diagram and note how many factors are inherently economic rather than related to the environment or health system.

Obesity: should the government intervene?

Recent estimates of the total costs of obesity, to the health care system and the wider economy (e.g. productivity) in England, range from about £6 billion to £20 billion per year. Even this enormous cost, however, may not justify government intervention (e.g. legislation or taxation against unhealthy practices, and subsidising or promoting healthy ones). Economists argue that when markets for goods (such as for healthy food, unhealthy foods, or exercise) do not produce outcomes that are desired by a society, they are said to 'fail' (see also Chapter 32 on 'perfect markets'). Below we describe two important types of market failure which may justify the intervention of governments in the relevant markets affecting the obesity problem: externalities and imperfect information.

Externalities

If an individual bears the full costs of their buying decisions (e.g. fast food), or behavioural choices (e.g. exercising less), then there are no external effects or **externalities**. If people do not bear the full cost, and some costs are borne by society more widely (e.g. by a collectively financed health system – see Chapter 34), then people will generally consume more or less of a good than is optimal for society as a whole. Through taxation on goods, governments can sometimes imitate the higher price that a good should have, and therefore reduce consumption to a level which reflects all of its impacts.

Imperfect information

Markets work best when both buyers and sellers are fully informed about the costs and benefits of goods or services being exchanged. In relation to obesity, imperfect information may exist if consumers do not know the calorific content of different foods, the amount of daily exercise that is optimal, or the relationship between being overweight and health risks. If imperfect information is a major cause of obesity, then governments could intervene through regulation (e.g. food labelling) or the direct provision of information (such as communicating the risk of diabetes or heart disease from obesity).

(a) Variations in the balance between public and private health care

	Source of Financing: Public or Private?	
Which organisations provide the care?	**1.** Publicly (state) financed & Privately provided	**2.** Privately financed & Privately provided
	3. Publicly (state) financed & Publicly (state) provided	**4.** Privately financed & Publicly (state) provided

(b) Public and private health expenditure per person in different countries (2008 US$)

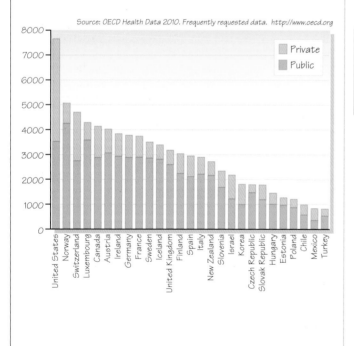

Source: OECD Health Data 2010. Frequently requested data. http://www.oecd.org

(c) Flow chart of finances in the German health system (circa 2002)

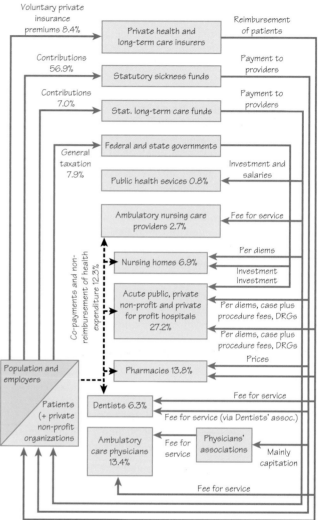

Sickness funds = the main bodies that provide compulsory health insurance in Germany. They are often regional rather than nationally based.

Fee for service = when doctors or hospitals are paid per item of care (e.g. per visit, per operation or per inpatient stay) usually according to an agreed schedule ('price list').

DRG = Diagnostic Related Group - a classification of similar items of care (similar resource use), usually for hospitals, which is used as a basis for fee for service payment. Used in many health care systems.

Per diem = a way of calculating care costs based on the number of days that a patient spends in hospital. Ambulatory care physicians - non-hospital based doctors, who in most countries would be primary care physicians (general practitioners) with no specific medical specialty.

Source: Busse R, Riesberg A. Health care systems in transition: Germany. Copenhagen: WHO Regional Office for Europe. 2004.
See further reading for reports describing other health care systems

Public Health and Epidemiology at a Glance, First Edition. Margaret Somerville, K. Kumaran, Rob Anderson.

In most countries the provision of doctors and other health professionals, and of the hospitals and clinics in which they work, involves national organisation, regulation and financing. This need to have a linked and coordinated 'national health care system' stems from the inevitable need for some government involvement in health care, which in turn stems from the different types of market failure from which health care generally suffers (see Chapter 31). Even in countries like the USA, where health care organisation is highly fragmented and dominated by private interests, the safety net of federal government and State-funded care programmes, plus the regulation of the insurance industry and the health professions, mean that it is still very much a publicly subsidised and government-regulated system.

'Public' versus 'private'

The organisation and financing of health care is often characterised using the polar opposites of 'public' (i.e. government control or ownership) and 'private' (non-government). In fact, the wide variety of health systems that exist shows that there is considerable variation between these two extremes, and that publicly financed health systems (e.g. by taxation) may provide most of their care through private organisations. Conversely, though less commonly, privately financed health care may be provided through organisations (e.g. hospital groups) which are publicly owned and run. There thus exists a spectrum of arrangements in terms of the degree and type of government involvement (see Figure 35a). Within the 'private' health care sector too, organisations may be for-profit or not-for-profit (e.g. charitable insurance funds or hospitals).

Who pays for health care and how?

Everyone pays for their health care by one route or another – varying from paying up-front and per episode of care ('privately'), through to various forms of optional private insurance, compulsory national health insurance or general taxation financed public provision. Because the need for health care is so unpredictable, and because the cost of care can be so expensive for individuals or families, people usually pay for health care collectively via some kind of insurance – either compulsory (usually state organised or regulated) or voluntary.

In countries like the UK, national health systems have emerged in which the government is both the main funder (via general taxation) and also the dominant provider of health care (quadrant 3 in Figure 35a).

Government financed and provided health care

In the UK and many Nordic countries health care is largely funded by general taxation. To a great extent the care is also provided by government-employed clinicians working in government-owned and managed hospitals and clinics, albeit through devolved local organisations. The main advantages for patients of such health systems are that they provide genuinely universal access to care (based on residency status or citizenship), and low or no co-payments for care (i.e. most care is free at point of use, regardless of ability to pay). They are also believed to be more amenable to reform, allow greater control of overall costs, and have lower administration costs than insurance-based health systems. Conversely, it is also argued that government funded and managed health systems may be unresponsive to patient or public demands, subject to more political interference, and be reluctant to innovate.

Social health insurance based systems

In many other countries in north-west Europe – such as Germany, France and the Netherlands – and also in Latin America, health care is primarily funded through compulsory social insurance. Like government-financed health systems, compulsory health insurance also ensures near-universal access to affordable care, but with the supposed advantages of better choice and responsiveness to public preferences and sometimes better-quality care. However, these advantages may come at a price. The disadvantages of social health insurance-based systems are that there may be variation in benefits for different categories of people (e.g. the employed and unemployed, or public sector and private employees), high administration and overall costs, and they are probably less amenable to reform than systems financed and provided by national government (Figure 35c shows the large variety and number of organisations in the German health system). High levels of 'co-payment' for care (that is, out-of-pocket charges to deter over-use of services) may also affect access to care for low income groups, even though voluntary insurance is sometimes encouraged to protect against these extra costs.

Private health insurance based systems

In the USA planning for the potential cost of illness and health care is historically an individual and family responsibility, so private health insurance forms the basis of health care funding. Insured people will typically pay for health care out-of-pocket but be partially reimbursed by the insurance company. However, private health insurance has failed to provide affordable health care for all. In particular, large proportions of the US population, especially children and the poor and unemployed, are either uninsured or 'under-insured' (i.e. they only have partial cover, for a limited range of acute care benefits).

The growth in the total cost of health care to the US economy is attributed to the incentives within private health insurance for over-provision relative to need. The insurance premiums have thus grown and become unaffordable (to both individuals and their employers). For these reasons, various publicly funded insurance and 'safety net' health care programmes have evolved – such as MedicAid and MediCare – for those on low incomes and the elderly, or for military veterans. Together these supplementary publicly-funded programmes mean that the US Federal and State governments spend as much public money per capita on health care as many countries whose health systems are almost wholly government-funded (see Figure 35b). In the 1990s, concerns about rising health care costs led to the growth of health maintenance organisations (HMOs), which serve defined populations with a standard package of subsidised care, often from a more restricted range of care providers.

Summary

National health systems are extremely diverse in terms of how citizens pay collectively to cover the cost of care, how universal any insurance system is, and therefore whether ability to pay affects the receipt of care. The consequences of these public and private financial and organisational arrangements are profound, for the autonomy of medical professionals, for the balance of investment in preventative programmes versus treating disease, and for the accessibility and responsiveness of health services to patients' needs and wants.

(a) The planning cycle

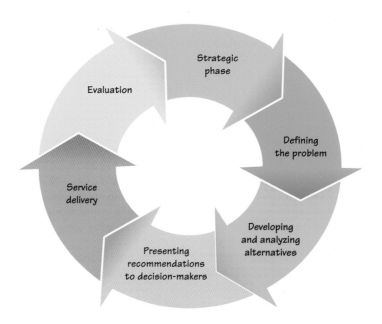

(b) Health equity audit

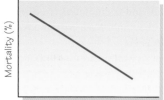

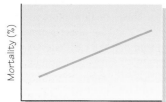

	If a service is equitably provided, then we would expect that the greater the need for health care, the more health care is provided. To check that services are equitable, health service use must be compared to some estimate of need for health care
	Need for health care could be represented by death or prevalence rates for a particular condition broken down by age, group, gender, geographical location or deprivation category
	Measure of health service use could be represented by treatment rates of the same condition – either drugs or surgical procedures
	In the upper graph, the red line shows an unfair service, where the greater the need for health care, the lower the health service use, while the lower graph shows health service use increasing with increasing need – a fair or equitable service. The relationship can also be expressed as a need: use ratio
	When Plymouth PCT carried out a health equity profile for coronary heart disease, they found that the mortality rates from CHD in the most depreived ares of the city were double those of the least deprived areas. While the emergency hospital admissions for angina and myocardial infarction showed the same gradient, revascularisation rates did not, providing evidence of inequity

Public Health and Epidemiology at a Glance, First Edition. Margaret Somerville, K. Kumaran, Rob Anderson.

A plan or a policy is an authoritative written statement of intent to aim for certain goals, to make certain organisational changes or to commit resources to particular types of activity. Such plans or policies may also include details of how these commitments are to be implemented. Planning, of health services or for any other type of large organisation, is the process of developing and disseminating such plans or policies.

Planning processes usually imply a rational approach to policy making whereby each stage of the planning process feeds into the next:
• Problem description leads to
• Formulation of goals and objectives, which lead to
• Specification of alternative possible actions, and then
• Choosing amongst those alternatives

Many descriptions of the planning process also include the essential stages of implementation and evaluation. Given that evaluation stimulates reassessment of the original problem, and a judgement about the success of the current plan, the outlined process can be defined as an iterative process, or **planning cycle** (Figure 36a).

Once the population need for health care has been understood, and the evidence assembled of what the effective interventions are for that particular need, then planners can ensure services have the right workforce, provide the effective interventions, are in the right place and have the capacity to cope with the expected workload. At least, that is the theory, but in practice many other considerations may influence the outcome of planning. Changing services to meet need takes time. Public and political views on the provision of health care may not match the public health view.

Equity
Public health is concerned with meeting the health needs of the whole population, not just those who are most able to reach or use services. When planning health services, therefore, explicit consideration must be given to ensuring that everyone who can benefit from a proposed service is able to receive it. It has long been recognised that those most in need of health care are least likely to receive it: this **inverse care law** was first articulated by Julian Tudor Hart, a GP in South Wales. For this reason, health services should be regularly monitored to ensure that they are equitably provided.

Figure 36b shows the principle of health equity audit, which compares need for health care with use of a health service or intervention. In the case of revascularisation described, mortality rates from coronary heart disease were used as a measure of need and revascularisation as a measure of health service use. For a service to be equitable, the expected relationship would be to note that the higher the mortality rate in a population group, the higher the revascularisation rate in the same group, but in the example quoted, this was not the case, suggesting an inequitable service provision.

Types of health service planning
Health service planning can occur at many different levels and can differ in terms of how plans are developed. Plans may be:
• National (e.g. whole health system) regional, local or hospital level

• Strategic (mainly about broad goals and general approaches to achieving change) or operational (about the specifics of organisational relationships and how to use resources)
• Evidence-based or more political in terms of the process of their development.

Some types of planning for health services may deal with specific problems or types of resource. For example, workforce planning (how many doctors and nurses will a country need to train during the coming decade?) or bed planning (how can the best use of available hospital beds be made during a winter influenza epidemic?)

Needs and evidence-based planning
Health services have often historically developed through incremental increases in resources: that is, existing services have been expanded by a certain amount each year. Political concerns and local and vested interests have also led to health services being developed differently in different local areas (e.g. the dominance of acute and specialist services in major cities). While there may have been good reasons for the initial establishment of such services, over time, changes in population and disease profiles may mean that services no longer meet the requirements of the people they serve.

The public health approach to planning is based on assessing the population need for a particular service. Needs assessment methods have already been considered in Chapter 21. Assessing the evidence of effectiveness of proposed interventions and services is an integral part of needs assessment; evidence may come from clinical trials or any of the other types of study discussed in Chapters 2–12, as well as local audits, evaluations and surveys.

Targets and monitoring
Targets are numerical policy goals, and often feature in national plans related to health. Examples include:
• Target levels of child immunisation in a population (e.g. in order achieve herd immunity)
• Target reductions in levels of road accident deaths
• Target levels of screening in specific population groups.

Some targets are related to public health outcomes, but may focus on process measures such as waiting times for treatment.

Clearly, to be effective, targets need to be monitored and also usually need a date by which the target should be met. Targets need to be realistic, yet also not be so easily achievable that they will not stimulate greater effort and innovation related to the ultimate goal of the policy. Ultimately the incentive for meeting targets depends upon the possible rewards or sanctions for meeting (or not meeting them) within the required timeframe.

Setting smoking cessation targets
In 2002, the Department of Health in England set a national target for smoking cessation services to reduce the prevalence of smoking by 800 000 smokers during 2003 to 2007. The target was measured as smokers who had successfully quit smoking for 4 weeks and it was to be achieved over a 3-year period. Each local area received an allocation from the 800 000 that was their contribution to achieving the national target, with intermediate targets set to ensure they were making progress.

37 Health care evaluation

(a) Main criteria used for evaluating health services or programmes

Criteria	Definition
Effectiveness	**Whether and to what extent a treatment or health service achieves its intended goals.** For treatments this will typically be some standard measures of *clinical effectiveness* such as the relief of symptoms, the reversal of disease processes, or survival. Health service effectiveness will usually encompass both clinical and non-clinical outcomes (e.g. quality of life, or treatments provided)
Safety	**Whether a treatment or health service causes adverse (i.e. unwanted) effects or harms.** Even if adverse effects are very rare events, if they are severe (e.g. death of infants) they may alter how care needs to be provided
Efficiency	**Efficiency, or cost-effectiveness, is the ratio of inputs to outputs.** In health care cost-effectiveness is usually expressed as the ratio of additional costs or savings implied by a new or alternative treatment or service, compared with the additional health-related benefits (e.g. deaths averted or Quality-Adjusted Life-Years), compared with the older/ next best treatment option
Equity	**Whether a service or programme is judged as fair,** often in terms of who is able to access or benefit from it relative to need. For example, if people in equal need of treatment (e.g. same disease severity) have different access to treatment, then there is horizontal inequity. If people in greater need of treatment do not have correspondingly greater access to treatment then this is said to be vertical inequity
Accessibility	**Whether people or those in need of health care can access the care or services they need.** Very difficult to measure without good data on both the number and characteristics of people who access a service, and principles and data for defining who should use a particular service or receive a treatment
Quality	**Whether or not a service or care package achieves intended effectiveness, acceptable safety, and establishes adequate processes of care.** Definitions of quality of care vary considerably and are often broad. They will usually span both clinical and non-clinical perspectives on outcomes, and specify attributes of care processes as well as patient-relevant goals
Satisfaction	**The patient or service user's overall judgement and specific views on a service or a specific episode of care** (e.g. an appointment or hospital stay). Questions about satisfaction or dissatisfaction should usually be developed directly from patient's views of what determines good or poor experiences of health care

(b) Donabedian's framework for evaluating health care

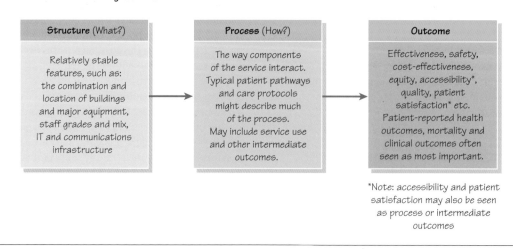

Structure (What?)	Process (How?)	Outcome
Relatively stable features, such as: the combination and location of buildings and major equipment, staff grades and mix, IT and communications infrastructure	The way components of the service interact. Typical patient pathways and care protocols might describe much of the process. May include service use and other intermediate outcomes.	Effectiveness, safety, cost-effectiveness, equity, accessibility*, quality, patient satisfaction* etc. Patient-reported health outcomes, mortality and clinical outcomes often seen as most important.

*Note: accessibility and patient satisfaction may also be seen as process or intermediate outcomes

Public Health and Epidemiology at a Glance, First Edition. Margaret Somerville, K. Kumaran, Rob Anderson.

Evaluation is the general term given to the assessment of whether something has achieved its intended goals or outcomes. More fully, it is the systematic, rigorous, and careful application of scientific methods to assess the design, implementation or outcomes of a programme, service or other defined endeavour. Organisations providing health services or public health programmes, funders, and service recipients all usually have an interest in knowing whether services are safe, effective and cost-effective.

Although it is sometimes seen as distinct from research, in practice some forms of research are also evaluation and vice versa. This includes the main clinical epidemiological study designs which aim to assess the effectiveness of treatments or programmes, such as randomised controlled trials. Furthermore, the principles of good evaluation are virtually indistinguishable from those of good research.

There are several main types of evaluation. **Outcome or effectiveness evaluation** aims to assess whether a programme is effective, economic evaluations consider whether a programme is cost-effective (see Chapter 32), and **process evaluations** assess whether the components of a programme function as expected and how they yield observed outcomes.

Evaluation criteria

Almost any activity, organisation or project can be evaluated against reasonable and measurable criteria. However, in health care a number of valued objectives have come to dominate. The main ones are:

- Effectiveness
- Safety
- Efficiency
- Equity (fairness)
- Access to care
- Quality of care
- Satisfaction or acceptability

These are all defined more fully in Figure 37a. Some of these can be measured for individual patients (e.g. effectiveness of a treatment, or patient satisfaction with a service) while others, such as equity or efficiency, can only be sensibly assessed at a whole service or community level. At the level of health services and health systems, other criteria might also be important such as responsiveness, or affordability.

Levels of evaluation: structure, process and outcome

In health care, three levels of evaluation are often specified: structure, process and outcome (see Figure 37b). Although this framework was originally developed by Avedis Donabedian for understanding the quality of medical care, the three-level typology of outcomes has influenced evaluation in health care more widely. Evaluating structure examines the provision of resources, facilities, equipment and staff to achieve particular goals. Evaluating processes, involves assessing how such human and physical resources are combined and used for those goals. Lastly, evaluating out-

comes simply involves measuring the attainment of the ultimate goals of the project or programme.

It is now seen as important to evaluate both process outcomes and final health and care quality outcomes together, usually within the same study. This recognises that most health care interventions are complex – they are multi-component, inherently behavioural (relying on the competence and motivation of providers, and the capabilities and adherence of patients) and context-dependent. Such complex health interventions and programmes will generally not be consistently effective (or cost-effective), so process evaluation enables some explanation of why health outcomes might vary from setting to setting and between studies.

Process evaluation often involves qualitative research methods, such as interviewing clinicians or patients, or observing how care is provided within a particular service. Qualitative research methods (such as interviews or focus group discussions) are especially important for documenting and explaining how patients experience care, or how doctors and patients interact and make choices during clinical encounters. Documentary analysis, for example studying the detailed content of policy documents, may identify the core concerns and main underlying concepts or assumptions used in designing services for particular groups of patients.

Audit versus research

In health care a key distinction between audit and research is recognised, mainly because research is believed to raise greater potential ethical concerns. In most developed countries, primary research involving data collection from or about human subjects has to go through a process of research ethics approval. In contrast, audit – the collection of data in order to assess whether an organisation's performance standards are being met – does not require research ethical approval. It also typically uses data that is already being routinely collected, to compare performance against standards or targets which have been set externally (e.g. see health equity audit described in Chapter 36). Clinical audit is defined as:

> quality improvement process that seeks to improve patient care and outcomes through systematic review of care against explicit criteria and the implementation of change (NHS – *Principles for Best Practice in Clinical Audit*, 2002).

Patient and public involvement

Health service evaluation has traditionally been conducted by clinicians, public health specialists or health service managers according to their service priorities and research interests. Today, however, patient and public perspectives are seen as paramount. In the 1990s a much greater emphasis was placed upon using patient-reported outcomes, such as health-related quality of life. More recently, there are also greater expectations of patient and public involvement in all stages of research and evaluation from survey design all the way through to the interpretation and dissemination of findings.

Self-assessment questions

Epidemiology and Evidence-Based Practice

1. Using Figure 2b, calculate the following:
   a. Incidence in the first year
   b. Incidence in the fifth year
   c. Point prevalence at the end of year 1
   d. Point prevalence at the end of year 4
   e. Period prevalence in the second year
   f. Period prevalence between years 3 and 5

2. Can you think of any factors which might explain why men in the areas shown in red on the map in Chapter 2 have higher than average deaths from mesothelioma?

3. As a junior hospital doctor in a district general hospital, your department is involved in a study examining the relationship between coronary heart disease and smoking. A case control study is performed. Cases are drawn from those admitted to the hospital with a primary diagnosis of CHD. Controls are inpatients of similar age and sex at the same hospital admitted for diseases other than CHD. Measurement of exposure (i.e. smoking) was obtained by a self-administered questionnaire. What is the most likely potential problem with this methodology?

4. You are interested in investigating whether exposure to high levels of radon increases the risk of developing lung cancer. Your study shows that people who live in high radon areas have a slightly higher risk of developing lung cancer. You also discover that the high radon areas have high deprivation scores. What is the most appropriate conclusion?

5. In a trial to examine the effectiveness of a new drug against standard treatment with oseltamivir (Tamiflu) in the treatment of swine influenza H1N1, subjects were randomly allocated to the two drugs through a computerised random number generator. What is the main advantage of randomisation?

6. In a large, randomised, double-blinded, multicentre trial testing the efficacy of clopidogrel 75 mg in preventing stroke, MI or vascular death in patients with clinical evidence of atherosclerotic disease compared to aspirin 325 mg (CAPRIE trial *Lancet* 1996;**348**:1329–39), the authors found the following results:
• Annual event rate (risk) of stroke, MI or vascular death in group given clopidogrel: 5.32%
• Annual event rate (risk) of stroke, MI or vascular death in group given aspirin: 5.83%
What is the number needed to treat (NNT)?

7. In the paper by Qin *et al.* Risk for schizophrenia and schizophrenia-like psychosis among patients with epilepsy: population-based cohort study (*BMJ* doi:10.1136/bmj.38488.462037.8F [published 17 June 2005]), the authors found the following relationship between a family history of epilepsy and the subsequent development of schizophrenia:
• Relative risk: 1.28 (95% C.I. 1.16–1.41) p<0.01
How do you interpret this result?

8. In a pilot study using faecal occult blood testing to screen for bowel cancer, the following results were obtained in a population of 100 000 people:

• 1950 tested positive, of whom 120 were subsequently diagnosed with bowel cancer after further testing.
• Of the 98 050 whose FOBT was negative, 50 were subsequently diagnosed with cancer.
• Calculate the prevalence, sensitivity, specificity, positive and negative predictive values and the positive and negative likelihood ratios for FOBT as a test for bowel cancer.

9. Which of the following options would reassure you that publication bias was not a significant problem in a systematic review and meta-analysis?
   a. The authors had included unpublished data from the manufacturers of the drug under investigation.
   b. The authors had searched the National Research Register for trials in progress.
   c. The funnel plot of included studies is symmetrical.
   d. The results of the meta-analysis do not show substantial heterogeneity.
   e. The authors analysed a subset of methodologically good trials.

Assessing Population Health

1. Deaths occurring in childhood contribute more to years of potential life lost than deaths over the age of 60. True or false?

2. Consider a population pyramid with a barrel shape in an imaginary country with a relatively small population (total population 10 million). A war breaks out, resulting in the death of a large number of young and middle-aged adults. What do you expect will happen to the shape of the population pyramid?

3. What would be the best data source for estimating the prevalence of rheumatoid arthritis in a defined geographical area?
   a. Referrals to the local specialist clinic
   b. Primary care records
   c. Death certificates
   d. Specific population-based survey.

Improving and Protecting Health

1. Classify the following actions as primary, secondary or tertiary prevention
   a. Screening for diabetic retinopathy
   b. Prescribing statins for a 55-year-old man with raised cholesterol levels and evidence of ischaemic heart disease
   c. Immunising children against the human papilloma virus
   d. Giving antiviral drugs to someone who has received a needlestick injury.

2. A new vaccine is being developed for a common infectious disease which affects people of all ages. The vaccine is due to be introduced nationally and administered to all age groups to eliminate the disease. The basic reproductive number for the disease is 4. What proportion of the population would have to be immunised to stop the transmission of the disease (assuming all the protection is from the vaccine alone)?

Health Economics

1. For each of the following economic evaluation methods, describe the type of unit in which benefits are measured:
   a. Cost-effectiveness analysis
   b. Cost-utility analysis
   c. Cost-benefit analysis.

2. In cost-effectiveness and cost-utility analysis, what is meant by *incremental analysis*?

3. If a group of patients receive treatment A, on average they live for 40 more years at a quality of life with a social preference weight (or 'utility') of 0.6. However, if they receive treatment B on average they live for only 30 years, but at a higher quality of life (utility weight of 0.9)
   a. How many quality-adjusted life-years (QALYs) are generated for a patient after each treatment?
   b. Which treatment, on average, produces the most QALYs?

Effective Health Care

1. Name the three main ways of financing health care, and name a country which exhibits each type of system.

2. Define the health system or health programme goals of *efficiency*, *equity* and *quality*.

Self-assessment answers

Epidemiology and Evidence-Based Practice

1. a. 10% b. 0 c. 40% d. 30% e. 60% f. 40%

2. The HSE report from which this map is taken comments that 'areas with the highest excess of mesothelioma deaths in males tend to be those which contain ports and dockyards, further supporting the well documented link between mesothelioma and past heavy asbestos exposures in the ship-building industry.'

For a detailed interpretation of these and other results, including problems with interpreting the data, see the discussion section of the full report, available online at www.hse.gov.uk/statistics/mesothelioma.htm

3. Selection bias: Selection bias is a potential issue in case-control studies. This can be minimised by ensuring that the controls are drawn from the same population as the cases. An ideal control is someone who would have been selected as a case if s/he had the outcome of interest.

4. The relationship between radon and lung cancer may be confounded by socio-economic deprivation. A confounder is a factor that is associated with both the exposure and the outcome and may be an alternative explanation for the findings.

5. It minimises confounding. If confounding is minimised or eliminated, then we can be more confident that any difference in the outcomes is due to the intervention and not due to other factors.

6. 196. Number needed to treat (NNT) is calculated by taking the reciprocal of the absolute risk difference (ARD)

$ARD = 5.83\% - 5.32\% = 0.51\%$

$NNT = 100/0.51$ or $1/0.0051 = 196$

7. Those with a family history of epilepsy have a 28% increased risk of developing schizophrenia. We are 95% confident that the true increase at population level lies between 16% and 41%; the probability of obtaining a result of this magnitude due to chance alone is less than 1 in 100.

8. Constructing the 2×2 diagram below is an essential first step before calculating the sensitivity, specificity, predictive values and likelihood ratios. Note the importance of getting the table the right way round, with the disease presence and absence in the vertical columns and the test results running horizontally.

Prevalence = 0.17%; sensitivity = 70.6%; specificity = 98.2%; PPV = 6.6%; NPV = 99.9%; LR positive = 39; LR negative = 0.3

9. a. T b. T c. T d. F e. F

		Bowel cancer		
		pos	neg	
FOBT	pos	120	1830	1950
	neg	50	98000	98050
		170	99830	100000

Assessing Population Health

1. T

2. The shape becomes 'hour glass' The death of a large number of young and middle-aged adults will affect the middle of the pyramid and result in a constriction there, while the upper and lower ends remain broad in the short term.

3. d. Referrals to a specialist service will depend on many factors, such as waiting times, awareness of the service by referring doctors and the criteria the service may set for accepting referrals (e.g. severity, nature or duration of symptoms). Primary care records are likely to be very variable in their completeness, but can be useful if there is good coverage of the population in the area, consistency of data recording and case definitions. As rheumatoid arthritis has a low death rate, death certificates will give a very low estimate of prevalence. Only a specific population-based survey is likely to give an accurate estimate, and then only if the methodology includes an adequate and well-designed sample of the population and clear consistent and objective criteria are used in the case definition.

Improving and Protecting Health

1. a. Although screening is usually considered secondary prevention, in this case the screening will not ameliorate the established disease of diabetes, but is aimed at reducing the effects of a complication of diabetes, namely retinopathy. Consequently, diabetic retinopathy screening can be considered tertiary prevention.

  b. Secondary prevention

  c. Primary prevention

  d. Primary prevention as the drugs are aimed at preventing any HIV infection developing

2. More than 75%. As the reproductive number is 4, it is essential to ensure that more than 3 of every 4 in the population are immune so that transmission stops and the disease will eventually die out.

Health Economics

1. Cost-effectiveness analysis – clinical units (e.g. cases detected or life-years saved); cost-utility analysis – QALYs or DALYs; cost-benefit analysis – money (e.g. £ or $).

2. Incremental analysis compares the additional costs of one alternative compared with another, with the additional effectiveness of the alternative (e.g. a new treatment compared with an old one). It involves calculation of the ratio of incremental costs divided by the incremental effects.

3. a. 24 QALYs after treatment A, 27 QALYs after treatment B.

  b. B

Effective Health Care

1. Government financed or general taxation-based (e.g. UK, Sweden), social health insurance (e.g. France, Germany, Netherlands), private health insurance (e.g. USA).

2. See definitions in Fig. 37a.

Public Health and Epidemiology at a Glance, First Edition. Margaret Somerville, K. Kumaran, Rob Anderson.

Appendix: Practical issues in conducting epidemiological studies

Box 1 Investigating an outbreak of diarrhoea and/or vomiting

A wedding party was attended by 200 guests. Following the wedding meal, a number of people become ill with diarrhoea and/or vomiting.

The initial actions will involve speaking to the people who were ill to get some information about the illness, probably using a standard questionnaire. The initial questionnaire would provide descriptive data on the people who were ill and identify any common factors that may require further investigation. Descriptive data could include age, gender, geography, onset of symptoms, type of symptoms, and any common factors such as attending the wedding and eating the wedding meal.

Box 2 Case-control study to investigate an outbreak of food poisoning

We can calculate the odds ratio of exposure to each risk factor of interest in cases compared to controls. For example, if the exposure of interest is raw salad, and the distribution is as below:

	Cases	Controls
Ate salad	40	20
Did not eat salad	10	30

Odds of exposure in cases = 40/10 = 4
Odds of exposure in controls = 20/30 = 0.66
Odds ratio = 6 (approximately)
This suggests that those who became ill were more likely to have eaten salad items at the wedding compared to those who did not become ill.

Box 3 Cohort study to investigate an outbreak of food poisoning

We can look at the relative risk or risk ratio of developing the outcome for a particular exposure. If we stick to salad items as the exposure, and the distribution is as below:

	Food poisoning	No food poisoning
Ate salad	40	60
Did not eat salad	10	90

Risk of developing food poisoning in those who ate salad = 40/100 = 0.4
Risk of developing food poisoning in those who did not eat salad = 10/100 = 0.1
Relative risk = 0.4/0.1 = 4
i.e. those who ate salad had four times the risk of developing disease compared to those who did not eat it.

Public Health and Epidemiology at a Glance, First Edition. Margaret Somerville, K. Kumaran, Rob Anderson.
© 2012 John Wiley & Sons, Ltd. Published 2012 by John Wiley & Sons, Ltd.

An example of investigating an outbreak of food poisoning

Epidemiological studies are usually carried out to:
• Describe a disease and its pattern in a population
• Analyse risk factors which determine why some people are affected and others are not.

In this section, we will focus on some practical issues involved in epidemiological studies using an outbreak of food poisoning as an example.

Box 1 outlines the initial actions that would be considered including basic descriptive epidemiology. The next step would be to perform an analytical study to try and identify the cause of the outbreak. The key issue with an analytical study is to compare one group of people with another group to be able to draw any meaningful conclusions. For example, if we discover that 80% of all smokers end up with COPD, that would be a descriptive study. However, that finding by itself is not very helpful unless we were able to show that the percentage of non-smokers who end up with COPD is much lower – say 10%. If 80% of non-smokers also end up with COPD, then the finding that 80% of smokers develop COPD would be meaningless. It is therefore the comparison between two groups of people which gives a better idea of risk factors and association between exposure (smoking) and outcome (COPD).

For such a situation, there are two types of epidemiological studies that would be feasible – case-control and cohort studies.

Case-control study

A case-control study would involve selecting cases (those with the condition or symptoms) and controls (those without). One of the key issues with any case-control study (see Chapter 8) is to avoid or minimise selection bias, particularly in the selection of controls. The controls should necessarily be drawn from the same population as the cases. It is necessary to have a case definition to identify cases appropriately. Cases can be selected either on the basis of clinical and epidemiological features with or without microbiological confirmation.

Going back to the illness outbreak at the wedding, a questionnaire specifically designed to cover the various likely exposures at the wedding will need to be administered to all cases and controls. The odds ratio of different exposure factors between cases and controls will help to examine the strength of association between each exposure and the condition.

Assume that 50 guests out of the total of 200 developed gastrointestinal symptoms and could be considered cases. The controls will have to be drawn from the same group that attended the wedding but were not cases themselves (i.e. an ideal control is someone who would have been identified as a case if s/he had the disease).

For pragmatic purposes, assume that we select one control per case. The questionnaire will need to identify all possible risk factors (based on the initial questionnaire given to cases). The questionnaire will have to be administered in exactly the same manner to cases and controls to minimise bias. It is important that cases and controls do not know which possible risk factors are being considered as potentially more likely to have caused the disease – otherwise those who have the disease will be more likely to remember a particular exposure (recall bias). It is also important that if the questionaire is administered personally, then the person administering it is not aware of the outcome, i.e. whether the person is a case or a control (to minimise observer bias). See Box 2 for a worked example of a particular exposure.

Cohort study

In a cohort study, we would need to select a cohort of people who would have had the opportunity to develop the outcome of interest – in this scenario, the wedding guests would form the cohort. We would then administer a questionnaire to the cohort collecting information about various exposures as well as information on illness.

Assume that all 200 guests form the cohort. As in the case-control study mentioned earlier, it is important for the measurement of exposure and outcome to be conducted as accurately as possible and in the same manner to minimise bias. The analysis will involve examining individual exposures and assessing the risk of developing disease. See Box 3 for a worked example of a particular exposure.

Statistical analysis

In both types of study design, the statistical analyses will include the conduct of significance tests and estimation of confidence intervals. A related issue is sample size, which has implications in epidemiological studies. Sample size calculations are ideally done in advance. They are based on the effect size we would like to detect, the significance level, and the power (the probability of determining a statistically significant result if it truly exists) for the study, and require expert advice. The details of sample size calculation are not discussed here, but it is important that the study is of adequate size relative to the aims of the study, such that an effect that is of clinical significance will also be statistically significant. It is important to be aware that a large sample size can produce a statistically significant result for a small effect and, conversely, even large effect sizes may not be statistically significant if the sample size is small. This has resource implications, too – an undersized study can be a waste of resources for not having the ability to detect important findings, while an oversized one may use more resources than required.

Further reading

General

Donaldson. L.J., Scally, G. *Donaldsons' Essential Public Health*, 3rd edition. Radcliffe Publishing, Milton Keynes, 2009.

Pencheon, D., Guest, C., Melzer, D., Muir Gray, J.A. *Oxford Handbook of Public Health Practice*, 2nd edition. Oxford University Press, Oxford, 2006.

Tulchinsky, T.H., Varavikova, E.A. *The New Public Health*, 2nd edition. Elsevier Academic Press, Burlington, MA, 2009.

UK Faculty of Public Health, www.fph.org.uk (accessed 05/12/11)

Epidemiology and Evidence-Based Practice (Chapters 2–11)

Bonita, R., Beaglehole, R., Kjellstrom, T. *Basic Epidemiology*, 2nd edition. World Health Organization, Geneva, 2006.

Cochrane Collaboration, http://ukcc.cochrane.org (accessed 05/12/11)

Coggon, D., Rose, G., Barker, D.J.P. *Epidemiology for the Uninitiated*, 5th edition. BMJ Books, London, 2003. Centre for Evidence-based Medicine www.cebm.net (accessed 05/12/11)

Critical Appraisal Skills Programme, http://www.casp-uk.net (accessed 28/12/11)

An Overview of Common Epidemiological Terms. Factsheet No. 5, South West Cancer Intelligence Service, www.swpho.nhs.uk (accessed 05/12/11)

Porta, M. (ed.). *A Dictionary of Epidemiology*, 5th edition. Oxford University Press, Oxford, 2008.

Straus, S.E., Richardson, W.S., Glasziou, P., Haynes, R.B. *Evidence-Based Medicine: How to Practise and Teach It*, 3rd edition. Churchill Livingstone, Edinburgh, 2005.

Assessing Population Health (Chapters 12–21)

Association of Public Health Observatories, www.apho.org.uk (accessed 05/12/11)

Costello, A., Abbas, M., Allen, A., *et al.* Managing the health effects of climate change. *Lancet* 2009;373:1693–733

Fair Society, Healthy Lives. Strategic Review of Health Inequalities in England post-2010. The Marmot Review 2010, www.instituteofhealthequity.org (accessed 05/12/11)

Global Health Risks 2009 www.who.int (accessed 05/12/11)

International Classification of Diseases, www.who.int (accessed 05/12/11)

Health Survey for England, www.dh.gov.uk (accessed 05/12/11)

An Introduction to Health Care Needs Analysis, http://www.hcna.bham.ac.uk/ (accessed 05/12/11)

Office for National Statistics, www.statistics.gov.uk (accessed 05/12/11)

Tackling Health Inequalities: A Programme for Action. Department of Health, London, 2003.

UK Association of Cancer Registries, www.ukacr.org (accessed 05/12/11)

US Census Bureau, www.census.gov (accessed 05/12/11)

World Health Organization, www.who.int (accessed 05/12/11)

Improving and Protecting Health (Chapters 22–30)

Hawker, J., Begg, N., Reintjes, R., Weinberg, J. *Communicable Disease Control Handbook*, 2nd edition. Blackwell Publishing, Oxford, 2005.

Health Protection Agency, www.hpa.org.uk (accessed 05/12/11)

Immunisation Against Infectious Disease (The Green Book), www.dh.gov.uk/greenbook (accessed 05/12/11)

Nutbeam, D., Harris, E. *Theory in a Nutshell*, 2nd edition McGraw Hill Australia, North Ryde, 2004

Otttawa Charter, www.who.int (accessed 05/12/11)

Raffle, A., Muir Gray, J.A. *Screening: Evidence and Practice*. Oxford University Press, Oxford, 2007.

Rose, G. *Rose's Strategy of Preventive Medicine*. Oxford University Press, Oxford, 2008.

Shapiro, S. Evidence on screening for breast cancer from a randomized trial. *Cancer* 1977;39(Suppl.):2772–82.

UK National Screening Committee, www.screening.nhs.uk, (accessed 05/12/11).

Health Economics (Chapters 31–34)

Drummond, M.F., Sculpher, M.J., Torrance, G.W., O'Brien, B.J., Stoddart, G.L. *Methods for the Economic Evaluation of Health Care Programmes*, 3rd edition. Oxford University Press, Oxford, 2005.

Mooney, G. *Economics, Medicine and Health Care*, 3rd edition, 2003. Prentice Hall, Harlow.

Propper, C. *Why Economics is Good for Your Health*. 2004 Royal Economic Society Public Lecture, CMPO, University of Bristol, http://www.bristol.ac.uk (accessed 05/12/11)

Effective Health Care (Chapters 35–37)

For comprehensive reports describing the organisation and financing of health care in different countries (*Health Care Systems in Transition* reports) go to the European Observatory on Health Systems and Policies, http://www.euro.who.int (accessed 05/12/11)

Index

abdominal pains 55
absolute risk differences 12–13, 25, 82, 84
   see also number-needed-to-treat . . . ; risk
      differences
absolute risks 12–13, 82, 84
   see also risks
accessibility criteria, health care evaluations
     80–1
active immunity 59
adverse effects, safety criteria 80–1
AF *see* attributable fraction . . .
affordability issues, economic evaluations 71
Afghanistan, health status measures 38–9, 44–5
African countries 34–5, 44–5
agents, disease transmission 51, 52–3, 54–5
ages
   see also inequalities . . .
   health status measures 38–9, 44–5
   population pyramids 32–3, 82, 84
   standardisation 18–19
aggregation bias 20–1
   see also ecological fallacy; information . . .
agriculture and food production, determinants of
     health 40–1, 43, 52–3, 69
air pollution, determinants of health 42–3
alcohol consumption 9, 17, 37, 39, 40–1, 48,
     50–1, 63, 74
   causal association 40–1, 48
   concepts 40–1, 48, 50–1, 63
   DALYs 41
   data sources 9, 37, 39
   HNAs 48
   interventions 48
   lifestyle determinants of health 40–1, 48
   liver cirrhosis 41
   oesophageal cancer 41
   sensible limits 41
Alcoholics Anonymous 48
analytical cross-sectional studies 21
antibiotic prophylaxis 55
antivirals, flu 24–5, 55, 82, 84
appendix 85–6
arthritis 37, 41, 82, 84
aspirin 82, 84
asthma 31, 71
asymptomatic infections 53, 60–1
attributable fraction (AF exposed) 38–9, 40–1
   see also causal association
attributable fraction (AF population) 38–9, 40–1
   see also causal association
audits and evaluations 8, 9, 78–9, 80–1, 83, 84
   see also evaluations
   definitions 81
   research contrasts 81
Australia, inequalities in health 45
availability issues, improving services 9, 78–9

barriers to public health 9
BCG 58–9
Beck's Depression Scale 31
bed nets 53
behavioural changes, promotion of health/well-
     being 64–5, 66–7

benzene exposure
   see also leukaemia
   risks 12–13
biases 15, 16–17, 20–1, 23, 27, 60–1, 82, 84, 86
   see also aggregation . . . ; causal associations;
     ecological fallacy; information . . . ;
     observer . . . ; publication . . . ; recall . . . ;
     selection . . . ; studies
   definition 17
   screening programmes 60, 61
   types 17, 23, 27, 86
biodiversity losses 42–3
biological-plausibility Bradford Hill criteria 14,
     15
birth rates, demographic transitions 33
blinding features of RCTs 24–5, 82, 84
blood tests 36
body mass index (BMI) 40–1
   see also obesity
booster doses 57
bowel cancer 61, 82, 84
Bradford Hill criteria 14, 15, 21
   see also causal associations
breast cancer 61, 62–3
breast-feeding initiation, data sources 36–7
British Paediatric Surveillance Unit 57
burden of disease, leading causes 72–3

cancers 12–13, 14–15, 16–17, 18–19, 36, 37, 41,
     42–3, 57, 60–1, 65, 71, 82, 84
   see also bowel . . . ; breast . . . ; cervical . . . ;
     leukaemia; liver . . . ; lung . . . ;
     oesophageal . . . ; prostate . . .
CAPRIE trial 82
car ownership 45, 74, 75
cardiovascular disease 17, 20–1, 34–5, 37, 39,
     40–1, 42–5, 72, 78, 82, 84
   see also coronary heart disease; strokes
   environmental determinants of health 42–3
   inequalities in health 44–5
   lifestyle determinants of health 40–1
Caribbean 44
carriage status, disease transmission 53, 55
case studies 14–15
case-control studies 12–13, 14–15, 22–3, 55, 82,
     84, 85–6
   see also observational . . .
   basic designs 22–3, 86
   cohort studies 22–3, 85–6
   critique 23, 86
   practical issues 85–6
Catholics, suicide rates 20–1
causal associations 14–15, 16–17, 22–3, 35, 38–9,
     40–1, 50–1, 65, 75, 82, 84, 85–6
   see also attributable fraction . . . ; Bradford Hill
     criteria
   alcohol consumption 40–1, 48
   cardiovascular disease 17, 21, 35, 40–1, 82, 84
   definition 15
   environmental determinants of health 40, 42–3
   lifestyle determinants of health 40–1, 65
   lung cancer 14–15, 16–17, 22–3, 41, 65, 82, 84
   obesity 40–1, 69, 74–5

smoking exposure 14–15, 16–17, 22–3, 39,
     40–1, 51, 65, 75, 82, 84, 86
census, data sources 9, 21, 30–1, 33, 34–5, 36–7,
     45
cervical cancer 71
chain of infection 52–3
chance occurrences 15, 16–17
   see also causal associations; confidence
     intervals; P values; studies
CHD *see* coronary heart disease
chemicals and poisons 8, 9
chickenpox 31
China, health status measures 38–9
cholera 53
cholesterol levels 40–1, 82, 84
chronic obstructive pulmonary disease (COPD)
     41, 42, 86
Clean Air Act 43
climate change 42–3
clinical audits, definition 81
clinical effectiveness, improving services 8, 9,
     48–9, 56, 57, 63, 80–1
clinical governance, improving services 8, 9
clinical roles of doctors and health services, public
     health contrasts 9
clopidogrel 82, 84
coastal reefs 42–3
The Cochrane Collaboration 27, 49
cohort studies 14–15, 22–3, 25, 55, 82, 84, 85–6
   see also nested case-control . . . ;
     observational . . .
   basic designs 22–3, 86
   case-control studies 22–3
   critique 23, 86
   definition 23
   experimental studies 25
   practical issues 85–6
collaborations, organisations 66–7
community actions
   diffusion of innovation theory 66–7
   promotion of health/well-being 64–5, 66–7
concealment-of-allocation features of RCTs 24–5
condoms 53, 55
confidence intervals 16–17, 26
   see also chance . . .
confirmed cases, surveillance 56–7
confounding factors 15, 16–17, 20–1, 23, 24
   see also causal associations; standardisation;
     studies
consistency Bradford Hill criteria 14, 15
consultations, data sources 9, 31, 36–7, 52–3, 82,
     84
contact factors, disease transmission 52–3, 54–5
contaminated fomites, routes of transmission 53,
     55
contaminated surfaces, disease prevention 53, 55
continuous data 28–9
continuous source epidemics 54–5
control policies, smoking exposure 64–5, 79
control principles, disease transmission 53, 54–5
controls, epidemiology definition 11, 86
convenience foods, obesity 74, 75
COPD *see* chronic obstructive pulmonary disease

Index compiled by Terry Halliday